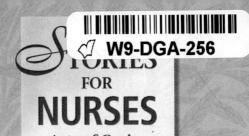

STORIES
FOR
NURSES
Acts of Caring

$\mathscr{S}$TORIES
FOR
NURSES
Acts of Caring

K. LYNN WIECK, RN, PhD
Associate Professor and Director of Research
Texas Woman's University
Houston, Texas
President, Texas Nurses Association

M Mosby
An Affiliate of Elsevier Science
St.Louis London Philadelphia Sydney Toronto

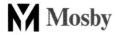

Mosby

An Affiliate of Elsevier Science

11830 Westline Industrial Drive
St. Louis, Missouri 63146

STORIES FOR NURSES: ACTS OF CARING

ISBN 0-323-02021-6

Vice President and Publishing Director, Nursing: Sally Schrefer
Acquisitions Editor: Yvonne Alexopoulos
Senior Developmental Editor: Melissa K. Boyle
Publishing Services Manager: Gayle May
Project Manager: Stephanie M. Hebenstreit
Designer: Teresa Breckwoldt

KI/B

Printed in the United States of America.

Last digit is the print number: 9 8 7 6 5 4 3 2 1

This book is dedicated to
the nursing students of this world
who are so anxious to capture that special
feeling of being a nurse. May you always
remember the excitement and the joy of
answering that noblest of callings,
being a registered nurse.

INTRODUCTION

Welcome to *Stories for Nurses: Acts of Caring*. This book is about the strength and resiliency of nurses. The strengths and achievements of nurses are often overlooked in the politics and chaos of modern healthcare. They shouldn't be.

This book is an acknowledgment of the realities of nursing and a challenge to make nursing better. The aim is to remind nurses why they became nurses in the first place and to rekindle that spark of enthusiasm. In the hectic pace of modern healthcare, it is easy to forget the happy moments, the triumphs, the joy of nursing. This book will shamelessly celebrate the positive side of nursing.

New nurses can glimpse the challenges they will face and identify strategies to manage and control their professional lives. Mid-career nurses can recapture the feeling of commitment and confidence that tends to get lost in the daily management of tasks. And senior nurses can remember all of the blessings that patients bring to the lives of nurses.

The sad and the happy sides of nursing are shared. Many of the daily routine tasks of nurses are presented in a different light. The usual becomes unusual, the everyday becomes special. Various points of view are offered, with an emphasis on the contributions and differences nurses make in the lives of the public we serve.

Finally, a positive future for nurses is proffered with a vision and a plan for the progress of nursing over the next 20 years. Read, enjoy, reflect, plan! The future is ours.

K. Lynn Wieck, RN, PhD

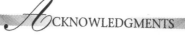

I wish to acknowledge the people who made this book possible. I want to thank the *Houston Chronicle,* the daily newspaper for the city of Houston, Texas, who originally published these chapters as columns in their healthcare supplement, "Health Care Professional Update." Their willingness to give a forum for promoting the positive side of nursing to over 40,000 nurses is so deeply appreciated. I also want to thank the many nurses and nursing students who shared their stories with me over the years. My gratitude goes to Yvonne Alexopoulos of Mosby for her immediate and unstoppable support of this project. And finally, the most important person in the evolution of this book was Alice Adams, *Houston Chronicle* editorial expert, who looked at these chapters with the practiced eye of a consumer and the expertise of her many years in journalism. She made them fun to read.

CONTENTS

SECTION I
A NOSE FOR NEWS

SECTION II
EXTRA, EXTRA, READ ALL ABOUT IT!

Section III
ALL THE NEWS THAT'S FIT TO PRINT

Section IV
NEWSFLASH!

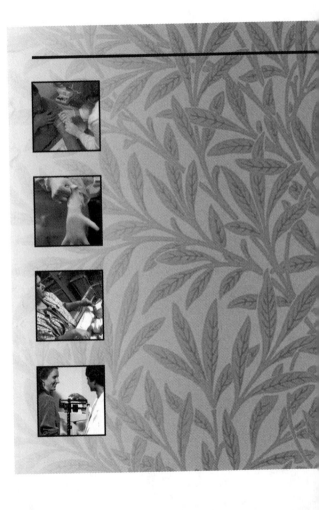

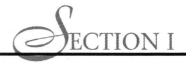
A NOSE FOR NEWS

*N*urses have that intuitive ability
to know just the right thing to say or do
to make patients feel better about things.
This section deals with nurses' sixth
sense, intuition, which puts the human
side into nursing. That ability to reach
out and touch people, to know the right
thing to say or do, to make a difference
in people's lives is what makes nurses
such special people.

CHAPTER 1

THE JOY OF NURSING

I love being a nurse! I'm not ashamed to say it. Nursing brings me joy every day of my life.

However, one of the concerns I have for both the current and the future workforce in nursing is the rampant amount of negativism. It seems that not enough positive things are being said about the nursing profession these days.

When you read about nursing in most newspapers and in magazines, the focus is mainly on how managed care is ruining everything. The healthcare picture portrayed in public media is usually very negative.

So, who is talking about the joys of being a nurse? If everything we read depicts the sorrows and horrors of nursing, can we expect to attract bright and dedicated young people into our profession?

It is past time for someone to talk about the joy of nursing.

True, there are a lot of days when nurses probably live closer to the negatives of managed care than the joys of being a nurse. When you are tired, overworked, underappreciated, and fearful for your license, it can be difficult to remember why you became a nurse in the first place.

Let's begin by talking about that "feeling." You know the one I am talking about?

It's that feeling you get when you reach deep inside your professional nurse self and do something that lights up the whole room. Maybe you are the only one who sees it. Maybe a patient, family, or peer sees it. Maybe the whole unit sees it. The important thing, however, is that **you** see it. You know when you do well, when you make a difference.

You also must know that sweet feeling deep in your inner self that flashes like electricity into your fingertips and your toes and makes you feel lighter than air. It's that feeling that spreads to your brain where a slight smile cannot be repressed, and you fear your whole head must be glowing like a neon sign in the darkness.

Then you look back at what you did, and you know you made a difference. You know it was extraordinary, and you savor the moment with this thought: "This is why I wanted to become a nurse!"

I think nurses are blessed with this feeling, although I imagine engineers get it, too, when their gadgets actually work. Maybe accountants get it when column A actually equals column B. I imagine teachers get it when a student finally grasps a concept or figures out a problem. But in nursing, we are so fortunate that incidents which trigger the feeling come often and leave us feeling invincible.

Remember when that patient crashed? You looked at the situation and knew just what to do with precision and compassion. Maybe a student or two were watching in awe and admiration. Your actions made a difference in a person's life. What an awesome privilege!

This special feeling is the essence of the joy of nursing.

I had one of those feelings recently when a perfect stranger came up to me and said, "You don't know me. I'm a nurse. I hated my job and had decided to get out of nursing recently, but I read your column [titled] 'My Most Unforgettable Patient,' and I remembered why I became a nurse. I decided I could never give that up, so I changed jobs, and I'm so much happier."

I thanked her for her kind words and continued along my path, as did she. But I kept wondering whether people were noticing the sudden brightness from my glowing head, or if they wondered what I was smiling about. It's that "feeling"! It's why I became a nurse.

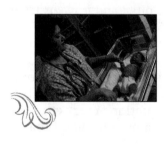

CHAPTER 2

SPONTANEOUS ACTS OF KINDNESS

A few years ago, a letter arrived at our home. It wasn't even addressed to me; it was for our son who was away at college. The return address was a home just down the street. Thinking our son had backed over someone's begonias again, I opened the letter to find out the damage.

The letter turned out to be a solicitation. One of my neighbors was chairing the Leukemia Society drive in our neighborhood and wanted to know if we would donate. I was so relieved that her begonias were still intact that I decided to write a check right then and there. I slapped the

7

modest check into the return envelope she had included, attached a stamp which she had not included, and then paused for a moment.

I thought about how much we in health-care depend on people just like my neighbor to raise the funds to sponsor research for the elimination of diseases. I also thought about how busy I think I am and how glad I was that I was not in charge of getting donations. So, I grabbed a handy sticky note and a pen and wrote this small note.

"Mrs. X, I want to thank you for taking your time and energy to raise money in our neighborhood to fight leukemia. I am a nurse, and we get to see the good that the money you raise does in helping little kids who would have died just a few short generations ago. I know you have a lot of other things you could do, so I just want to tell you how much I appreciate you. Enclosed is my check to help this cause. In Admiration, Lynn Wieck."

The whole thing took less than a minute or two. I stuck the note to the check and sent the letter on its way. I didn't even take the check to her; I let the mail carrier do the leg-work. I never gave it another thought.

A few weeks later, I received a call in the early evening hours. The voice asked to speak to me. I immediately went into my "anti–phone-solicitor" mode, but she informed me she was my neighbor. Figuring *I* had creamed someone's flowers this time, I switched to my "sorry—it was an accident" mode. Here's what she said:

"I just moved to this community a few months ago. I am retired and have been doing solicitation drives for several charities for over 18 years. I just want you to know how much I appreciate your note. In 18 years, that is the first time anyone ever thanked me for asking them for money."

We had a nice chat—short, friendly, uplifting. When she hung up, I knew she felt good. I felt good. The endorphins were raging. There was happiness in the air. And I thought about how this spontaneous little act had triggered something so good.

What do you think Mrs. X believes about nurses based on this incident? I hope she thinks they are nice, kind, polite, mannerly, and grateful. When Mrs. X's extremely bright and gifted granddaughter comes for Christmas this year and says, "You know,

Grandma, I think I want to be a nurse," what do you think she'll say as she gazes at this darling child who is the light of her grandparent's eyes? Maybe she'll say, "Yes, dear, that sounds perfect for you."

Who knows? My point is that people remember things. They remember the nurse who was rude to them in the emergency room, the nurse who made them leave the ICU when Grandpa was so sick, the nurse who was too busy to pull the sheets tight so Johnny could sleep. So why wouldn't they remember nice things, too?

I share this story because I know that thousands of you perform this exact same type of spontaneous kindness every day. You probably think no one is watching and that no one cares. I beg to differ. Someone is always watching, and everyone cares. We have such a wonderful opportunity to sell our profession when we engage in spontaneous acts of kindness as nurses. Nursing attracts kind and generous people who care about others.

Life is in overdrive today. The pace is fast, and if you slow down, you might get run over. This chaos and frenzy is making us tired. It is also crowding out the little things we do that make such a big difference.

My biggest fear is that we will lose the energy and will to perform these spontaneous acts of kindness that make the public (as well as ourselves) feel good about nursing and about life itself. It would be terrible to cheat ourselves out of the pleasure that comes with being kind to others, even when no one is looking.

I want to be presumptuous enough to thank each of you for your spontaneous acts of kindness on behalf of all nurses. You make us look good. You make nursing an attractive career alternative. And, you contribute to your own sense of self-worth. Those huge benefits are worth a few minutes of our time any day.

CHAPTER 3

MILESTONES

Recently, my husband and I proudly watched as our third (and last) son graduated from college. As we sat in the huge auditorium packed with families and friends, I was struck by the significance of these types of events in people's lives.

Think back over the milestones in your life. A milestone is a significant event in a person's life history. I wonder how many of these milestones relate to your chosen profession.

When we think of significant events, we usually think of things like births and weddings. Completion of an educational program and receiving awards are also significant. Some milestones are not so positive, such as deaths and divorces, but we remember and celebrate our capacity to overcome sadness and to go on with our lives.

What are the hallmarks of a milestone? We usually take a lot of photos and have friends and family around us. An emotional response is involved, and the event is remembered and recalled, often for years to come. The best part is a feeling of accomplishment and satisfaction. In healthcare, however, our milestones are often more subtle.

Think about the milestones in your professional career. One would certainly be the completion of your education. Your graduation or pinning held a special moment of accomplishment and pride for you and your family.

Remember the feelings of relief and excitement as you entered your chosen career. Remember your uncertainty about being able to do the job well. How about your confidence that you could go out and fix all the problems that were plaguing healthcare—and your dismay at finding out what the real world was like? That milestone still brings back a lot of mixed emotions for me.

Do you remember your first real accomplishment as a new healthcare professional?

Maybe it was the first IV you started on a patient with impossible veins, the first time you had the instrument in the physician's hands before the word was even spoken, the family who came back to tell you how much your words and presence meant to them in a crisis.

During my first six months as a nurse on a urology unit, we had an overflow plastic surgery patient. The plastic surgeon, unhappy at having to visit a urology floor in the first place, stopped in the middle of a dressing change and complimented me on how well I had cut the gauze so it would not ravel and interfere with the healing of his tiny, precise stitches. For heaven's sake, he complimented me on cutting a straight line, but I felt like I had been awarded the Medal of Honor and still remember his words these 32 years later.

I had put the patient's needs ahead of my own busy schedule, and someone had noticed. What a great feeling!

What about your first patient death? That is a milestone for many of us. Do you realize how privileged we are to assist at people's deaths? Remember that first time one of your patients died, and the family looked to you for comfort and guidance? That was the time that you found out that you did, indeed, know what to say and whom to call. You could see the relief in the family's eyes that someone had control in a situation that they could not control. It was one of those wonderful, precious moments in nursing when you know you are needed and your actions ease the pain and suffering of another person.

Unfortunately, in the hectic chaos of healthcare today, it seems that the acknowledgment of milestones has gotten lost. We are so busy just trying to cope with the complex world that we do not have time to celebrate special moments. It is like treading water. We aren't sinking, but we aren't making a lot of progress either.

I strongly urge you to recognize the new discoveries in your own practice. Pat yourself on the back when you take a big step, or even a small one. Promotions, recognition, triumphs—we should all celebrate them because they are part of the special commit-

ment we have made to serve the health needs
of the public.

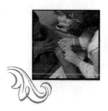

CHAPTER 4

THE OTHER SIDE OF PAIN

Illness, surgery, and recuperation can be painful experiences.

When thinking about patients in pain, something nurses see on a daily basis, the first thing I envision is all of the things we do to ease a patient's pain and suffering. It's not only a primary part of our professional role but also, as patient advocates, easing pain must be a commitment.

Thanks to the miracles of modern science, nurses have a lot of weapons to call on in our war against pain. We use assessment techniques to discover the extent of a patient's pain. Research shows the 1 to 10 pain scale (with 1 being no pain at all and 10 being the most pain you can imagine) to be a very good indicator of pain in adults. In children, we use the Wong Faces Pain Scale where children can point to the face that looks like their pain.

We use a wide variety of pain-inhibiting medications to stop or buffer pain. We use many other techniques, such as distraction therapy with children, meditation, and visual imagery to help patients manage their pain. Other comfort measures, such as a back rub, padding or elevating on pillows, and warm baths are also available to increase the patient's comfort.

As a group, nurses have become quite adept at managing patients' pain and increasing their comfort. But there is another side to pain.

As I wrote this commentary, I felt the need to immediately state this point—nurses never intentionally cause pain, but sometimes it just happens. At that moment, I realized the statement is not true. Nurses do, indeed, intentionally cause pain on occasion.

We make patients do things that we know, and they know, are going to be painful. For example, we make them get out of bed three hours after their return from surgery; we turn them in bed from side to side, even when patients have huge leg casts; and we make them do the unthinkable—take deep breaths and cough even with incisions all the way across their abdomens screaming at them to stop.

We ask, in fact, we *insist* that patients do a lot of things that result in pain.

So how do I reconcile this "truism" with my belief that nurses are the patient's advocate, the ones who stand up and assure that each patient receives proper care?

Do patients need pain? Of course not!

But we all realize the consequences of not getting out of bed, of not turning, and of declining to do deep breathing. And those potential consequences are more painful to us than causing some momentary pain.

The nurse's most important immediate role is to be sure that the patient has the full story about why the transient pain of the moment is necessary. After getting your one-thousandth patient up after back surgery to walk down the hall as ordered and expected, you might think that your patented little explanation of why this is all necessary is not worth delivering. After all, this enlightened healthcare consumer should understand why it is necessary to get up after surgery and what the threats are to the circulatory and respiratory systems.

When you are tempted to just skip the explanation and get on with the job, I would urge you to remember that all pain is personal. While I "knew" all about childbirth (I had been a nurse for six years), I can assure you that when it got "personal," I needed basic information just as much as any uninformed, first-time mom.

Bottom line, your one-thousandth explanation should be just as compassionate and sincere as your first one. Every patient deserves a caring and compassionate nurse, and for each encounter we should use our very best nursing judgment and actions.

So let's continue to try to alleviate pain to the best of our ability, especially when we are the cause of it. Be sure your patient understands why the action is necessary and how we are going to make it as easy as possible. Use prophylactic pain management whenever possible (e.g., giving the pain medication 30 minutes before the activity so the patient will receive optimal benefit). Never let a busy schedule or pressing needs get in the way of doing what nurses do best, advocating for each and every patient to ensure that they reach their optimal health goals as painlessly as possible.

CHAPTER 5

DEATH AND DYING—A PART OF NURSING LIFE

As nurses, we are often asked by our non-nurse friends about how we can stand to deal with such serious issues as life and death.

Although many nurses work in low-risk areas where the focus is on health promotion and maintenance, we do deal with end-of-life issues regularly. These issues are much more complex and harder to grasp. Why do nurses choose to work in settings where patients die? How does the experience affect nurses? It might be interesting to look at three different perspectives on the issue.

Perhaps the most difficult patient death for nurses to handle is one that occurs on the general patient unit. Some patients spend months and even years in this unit, where the nurses become like extended family. We get to know the patients and their families. However, because a hospital is a place for sick people and there is no sure cure for all illnesses, people sometimes die.

Nurses often attend funeral services for these deceased patients and act as a support to the family whom they came to know very well. This action is a benefit to both the family and the nurse.

The intensive care unit (ICU) is another area where nurses must confront death. Devastating, life-threatening injuries are a common part of the ICU nurse's day. The goal, of course, for all ICU patients is to regain health to the point that they can be discharged to the general hospital unit, recover, and go home. ICU nurses work diligently toward this goal of full recovery for all patients. The reality, however, is that ICU nurses become intimately familiar with the dying process. They accept that death is inevitable for some patients, and they acknowledge that death is a part of life. An ICU nurse once said, "We try to make the experience as painless as possible for both the patient and family."

Hospice nursing, a third area where nurses deal intimately with death, has as its focal point nurses who provide care and comfort for people who are in the final phase of life. In fact, a patient usually cannot be admitted to hospice unless he or she has accepted that death is imminent. The focus is on the quality of remaining life, pain management, and a peaceful death.

When asked how hospice nurses handle the certain outcomes of their patients, one hospice nurse said, "We cry, we laugh, we talk about it. We have strong support among ourselves."

Nurses are geared to both care and cure. Realizing that not every patient can be saved, nurses still have emotional reactions to understanding and accepting when a patient dies.

And yet, most nurses survive and thrive in their positions by focusing on the many triumphs that occur instead of the occasional unexpected problem. The joy of seeing a person make great strides, return to his or her life, conquer a health condition, or have a peaceful, joyous death certainly offsets any sadness that occurs in the everyday life of a nurse.

CHAPTER 6

NURSING PRESENCE

How do nurses deal with grief? I could not figure out why that question was posing such a problem for me. I should know the answer. I have been a nurse for 30+ years, and I know lots of nurses. Why couldn't I snap out a short, to-the-point response to that simple question?

The more I pondered how nurses handle grief, the more frustrated I became. Finally, it came to me. Nurses handle grief just like everyone else does. After all, nurses are people, too.

In grief, some of us cry, some of get angry, some of us hide from grief, and some of us feel let down or feel like a failure. I will wager that if you polled the world, you would find those are ways lots of people deal with grief.

But it has occurred to me that we as nurses do one thing in grief that is consistent with the caring and nurturing way we approach our chosen profession. I believe that nurses consistently use the gift of "presence" or "being there" to help the patient and family deal with grief. I have often heard or read notes from families after a death when they thank the nurse for "being there when we needed you most."

After the physician walks in and delivers bad news, who is left behind to be present with the patient during the struggle to absorb the devastating reality? After the clergy and the family have left for the day, who remains present for the patient after the words "metastasis" or "incurable" have been uttered?

Nurses know that just our presence can have a calming effect on people who are trying to deal with the unthinkable. Often we know that there is absolutely nothing we can do to change the diagnosis or the eventual outcome, but the consolation of having a nurse present, of having a nurse share the pain, of having a nurse care, can be one of the most therapeutic aspects of a patient's adjustment to bad news or a family's adjustment to the loss of their loved one.

I believe nurses have mastered the art of letting in the silence. We often do not need words. Many of us have carefully placed pillows under the shoulders and hips of dying patients even though we know that the morphine has made the use of pillows inconsequential—but the wife and children feel better that something is being done. Many of us have placed a wet cloth on parched lips of patients with Cheyne-Stokes respirations more to benefit the family than the patient. It is the silent presence of the nurse, "someone who knows what to do," that brings solace to a family frustrated because they don't know what to do.

Although many of our colleagues in medicine still see death as a defeat, as a failure, I believe nurses are better able to accept the inevitable. I wonder if that happens because we still have a patient. The family becomes our patient, and without missing a beat, we incorporate the family as patient during grieving situations. We use that therapeutic presence, often in silence, to let the family know they are not alone and that all that could have been done was, indeed, done.

We attempt to alleviate guilt, to soothe anger, to reinforce strength, and to acknowledge loss. It is a delicate time. How do we do it? By being there.

CHAPTER 7

SEXUALITY AND OTHER SENSITIVE TOPICS

During a conversation about health promotion in older people one day, the topic came around to sexuality, and how uncomfortable many nurses are in discussing it.

True, obstetrical nurses seem pretty comfortable talking about birth control, and public health nurses and school nurses are very good at talking about sexually transmitted diseases. But we noted that many hospital nurses still did not accept and practice routine screening and assessment for physical and sexual abuse in their patients. Although there is an excellent, short, nonjudgmental screen for physical and sexual abuse that has been available for over a decade now, you will have a hard time finding any nurse who uses it regularly. We wondered why.

In your practice, do you regularly screen for sexual abuse? Do you ask your patients if they have any questions about their physical or sexual health?

If you do, congratulations. If you don't, you are not alone. I think there is a great reluctance on the part of nurses to "cross the line." When is it therapeutic and when is it being "nosy"? Will the patient be intimidated or embarrassed? Will I be sued for sexual harassment?

Perhaps the best bet is to do what we do best—relate to our patients. We are experts on nonverbal cues. We can pick up a patient's anxiety before he or she ever says a word. We are alert to early signs of pain and know what to do about it. I am certain that we can discern whether our patients want or need to talk about sexual problems if we just give them a chance.

I am making the case that to deny a patient the opportunity to ask questions about sexual concerns is no different than denying the opportunity to ask about a new medication or how to change a dressing. We would not dream of sending a patient home with a central line unless we had explained it in detail, both orally and in writing. But we think nothing of sending an elderly woman home after hip surgery without any information regarding safe sexual positions.

I heard that little voice in your head say, "Oh my gosh, don't be disgusting. Old people should not be having sex anyway." That brings me to another point. I think that a young man who has an arthroscopy probably has no problem asking when he can "get romantic," and the nurse has no problem in telling him. But what happens when older people want to know about sex? Who do they ask? Sexual interest, activity, and needs are maintained well into old age, provided the person remains in good health and has an interested partner. There is no reason that people who have enjoyed a happy and satisfying sexual relationship cannot continue to do so into their sixtieth, seventieth, eightieth years, and beyond.

Conversely, consider this question—how did older people learn about sex? They learned by watching the farm animals and through trial and error. There was no HBO or MTV in the 1930s. So, while they may be fine receiving information about their medicine or their blood pressure from a person in a white coat, that is probably not the way they have learned about sex.

Sexual problems in the elderly commonly result from emotional and social factors rather than biological or organic conditions. Impotence has received a great deal of interest lately because of new drugs to treat it. However, most cases of impotence are a result of emotional rather than physiological factors. Often, just knowing the facts may mean the difference between a happy sexual life and no sex at all or feelings of frustration and failure.

If your patients do ask you about sex, I encourage you to be open to their questions. Some women may fear or be embarrassed by sexual enjoyment. A nurse's best tactic is to ask whether they have questions, to answer them honestly and openly, and to avoid any sense of judgment or shock. Some people are afraid they will have a heart attack and die during sexual intercourse. Reassure your patients that it is unlikely that they will die during intercourse with their usual mate and in friendly surroundings. In terms of energy expended, conjugal intercourse is comparable to climbing one or two flights of stairs or taking a brisk walk.

I hope all of us will be sensitive to the needs of our patients for information, especially the most vulnerable. Those who cannot get the information anywhere else are particularly dependent on the nurse. What most people need is factual, nonjudgmental information so they can make up their own minds whether or not to have sex. Nurses are trusted to answer questions without passing judgment. Thanks for caring for the total patient—you are the only ones who do.

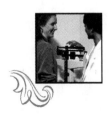

CHAPTER 8

NURSES' STORIES

Have you ever noticed how nurses talk to each other? Have you picked up on how we share our knowledge? When we want to teach, we often share personal experiences.

I believe that my Cherokee great-great-grandmother would have been so proud of me being a nurse; she would probably have been a nurse herself. Why? Because one of the beauties of the American Indian culture is that they speak in stories. It is becoming clear to me that nurses also speak in stories.

When we want to explain to students the concept of caring, we do not explain the mechanism of endorphin release when a certain receptor is triggered by a stimulus. We tell a story of an elderly patient who had no visitors and who died with a caring nurse holding his hand long after her required shift was completed. We tell about the time we sat in a small dark room and cried with a young woman who had just learned that she could never have the baby she and her husband so desperately wanted.

When we want to explain the concept of humor in nursing, we don't go into the physiological changes in the body when we laugh. We tell about the little old man who nearly ended up in ICU after he thought it would be amusing to put his apple juice in the urine specimen bottle, just to see if anyone noticed. We tell about the time that the elevator got stuck between floors on Thanksgiving day and the only person on board was the resident psychiatrist who could not really tell everyone when he finally got out how angry, upset, and scared he was during his ordeal. After all, he was a psychiatrist.

When we are discussing disaster nursing and the need to be prepared for emergencies, we do not recite a litany of supplies and equipment to have on hand. We tell about the time that the tornado swooped down on the trailer park next to the small lake. We tell about the panic of a man running all over town checking emergency rooms searching for his two children after a school bus accident. We tell about the day it snowed so much that the next shift could not get into the hospital; we had to work for 36 hours and then were taken home in the back of Army Reserve trucks with flapping sides and no heaters.

My friends are going to be surprised that I would write about stories. I do not much care for qualitative research, which to me is the attempt to discover knowledge about people and nursing by listening inquiringly to stories. I like numbers—if four out of five people have it, we need to do something about it. However, you cannot discount the fact that nurses have beautiful and meaningful stories to support many of these hard statistics.

Each of you has wonderful, and sad, stories to share. If you think about it, our lives are just a series of stories. Sometimes the stories have a happy ending and sometimes they don't. But nurses' stories must be the best in the world because, every day, we touch people's lives. Our stories are the stories of people at their very best and their very worst, of supreme triumph and abject loss. Cherish your stories. Share them with others. We need to attract bright young people into the nursing profession. One of our best recruitment tools is our large pool of beautiful stories.

CHAPTER 9

MY MOST UNFORGET- TABLE PATIENT

Every nurse has had that special patient who will be remembered forever. Regardless of the passage of time or the circumstances of the encounter, all nurses can tell you about their most unforgettable patients without any hesitation.

To reassure myself of this point, I posed this question to a colleague: "If I asked you about your most unforgettable patient, could you tell me?" In less than a second she responded, "Of course. I had just finished my shift in CCU, and she took my hand and begged me not to leave so she would not have to die alone. She had no family, so I stayed at her bedside all night until she died, just before daybreak. She never let go of my hand."

Your most unforgettable patient may bring up happy memories or sad ones, but one of the best things about being a nurse is the times you get to share with patients.

What other profession can boast about having the privilege of sharing the most intimate, the most critical, the most life-altering moments of their clients' lives? Do you ever hear accountants talk about their most unforgettable ledger sheets or bank tellers talk about their most unforgettable bank accounts? Probably not.

In healthcare, we are there when human beings experience those dynamic moments that make them human. We are there during birth, at the time of death, during pain and the relief of pain. We share life-altering decisions and body-altering treatments. We offer support, encouragement, and friendship. What a precious gift—to be able to share these most intimate and important times of our patients' lives.

But sharing critical moments means we also share the happiness, sadness, fear, frustration, anger, and helplessness of these emotional times. We see patients at their best and at their worst. And it is through these privileged insights that we can remember those unforgettable patients. It is also an important part of what makes our lives and our careers so interesting and so enjoyable.

I am not going to tell you about my most unforgettable patient. Instead, I would invite you to take a moment or two to remember your most unforgettable patient. Remember the emotions surrounding the encounter. Whether the experience was happy or sad, funny or embarrassing, gratifying or frightening, remember that every day a part of your professional life is spent making a difference in people's lives.

As you search your memory for those significant moments in your nursing career, rejoice that you have chosen a career that is built on being involved in the lives of others. Many people in this world go to work every day uninspired and unmotivated. They have jobs that earn them a living, but really don't make that much difference. They contribute their time, but they hold back their *selves*. They show up each day, but they never get involved. One of the joys of nursing is that it is not a spectator profession—you have to get involved.

This investment of your whole heart and soul is what makes you a special nurse. It is also what makes your patients special. As you remember that one patient who was most special, remember that he or she benefited from the fact that you decided to be a nurse.

There are many joys in being a nurse. Every day, you share your healing gifts with people who need you so much. I can only hope that one day when one of your patients is asked, "Tell me about your most unforgettable nurse," he or she will smile and, without hesitation, share a happy and healing moment spent with you.

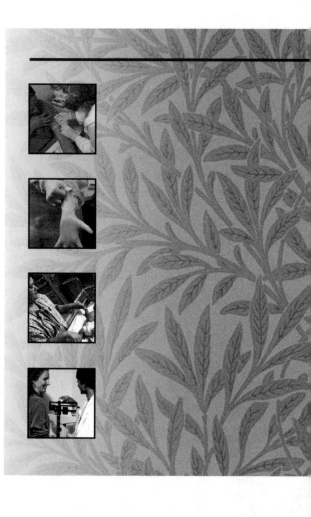

EXTRA, EXTRA, READ ALL ABOUT IT!

Much of the great news in nursing is how nurses take care of each other and themselves. Sometimes we are more successful than others. This section talks about the importance of nurturing ourselves and our nurse colleagues as we progress through our nursing careers. It is a lonely road to go alone. Focusing on what nurses like about nursing, what drew us into *nursing in the first place, and what keeps us in nursing are vital parts of the rejuvenation and appreciation process. Going the extra mile is what makes nurses special.*

CHAPTER 10

HUMOR IS GOOD FOR WHAT AILS YOU!

We've all heard it, but is laughter really the best medicine? Research has shown that one good, deep belly laugh per day is good for circulation, respiration, agitation, and probably constipation.

So if laughter is so good for us, why is it so rare?

Healthcare has been a great beneficiary of technological advancements. Many lives are saved each year because of the modern equipment, medicines, and techniques available.

So why aren't we happier about it? It appears to me that the mood in hospitals has grown increasingly somber.

Although I recognize that a hospital is not a comedy club, I believe the absence of laughter is not therapeutic or even healthy. What has happened? Where did all the laughter go?

I would like to propose a possible answer. Hospitals have always been serious business. People die there. Lives are changed forever in hospitals, and that has always been the case.

I invite you to walk down the halls of a hospital and count the number of people you see smiling or laughing. Nurses used to spread sunshine and cheer along with medicines and back rubs. I propose that the cheer has gone the same route as the back rubs. No one has time anymore.

"Oh, great," you are probably moaning, "One more thing for me to do—be a little ray of sunshine."

I know that your patients would benefit from an occasional smile, but my motives are not that pure. I am being terribly selfish. I think that a happy nurse is a healthy and more competent nurse.

Who do you want to administer your Coumadin dose—the nurse who is smiling and chatting with you about the small bruise on your ankle that has not gotten any bigger, or the nurse who is frowning while trying to remember all of the things to be done before shift change and who ignores the new bleeding on your bandage? Your choice.

I firmly believe we take ourselves too seriously in this world, especially in nursing. Try to differentiate between those times when seriousness is essential and when it is an unnecessary encumbrance.

While you are figuring out my medication dose or determining my IV rate, I want "serious." But when you are trying to decide who goes to lunch first or who will work the double shift to cover for a colleague who is ill, a little humor can be a wonderful ally.

Sick patients need to see a smile. They need to hear a laugh. Even if they cannot laugh themselves because of tubes or pain, they need the hope that laughter is not far away. Sometimes hope is all we can offer people. I believe that laughter and happiness are things worth hoping and waiting for.

So I urge all of you to have at least one good laugh per day. If you are really desperate, buy a humor book or an issue of *Reader's Digest*. Look at the humor in situations.

A glass is either half empty or half full—it just depends on how you look at it. Step back and make yourself take a deep breath before you snap at someone. Laugh at the absurdity of the situation and go forward. You will not only be a much sought-after ally by your coworkers, but you will also like yourself better, too.

Brighten up your world with some laughter and some cheer. Don't worry that you might miss some of the problems in healthcare; there will always be plenty of people anxious to point out what's wrong. What we need in nursing is more people pointing out what's right. It is wonderful to be a nurse. Enjoy yourself!

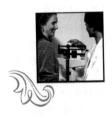

CHAPTER 11

CELEBRATING
EXCELLENCE
IN THE
WORKPLACE

Families play such an important part in our lives. When we are little, they provide us with a safe place to try new things, to make mistakes and still be accepted. As a child, everything we do is wonderful. We know because our families tell us so.

Our parents praised us when we took those first steps or said that first word. Our moms took the pictures we drew of the dog—whether we gave him three legs or all four—and hung them on the refrigerator. Then they called our grandmothers to tell them how smart we were. We basked in their praise.

When our dads took the training wheels off our bikes and we rode, alone, for the first time, they were as proud as we were scared. We celebrated these accomplishments. In turn, we now praise our kids. It builds their self-esteem. It adds to their feelings of importance, and it makes them feel good about themselves.

In school we also got feedback in the form of "grades." No matter how much we hated the tests, the grades were tangible proof that we had done something. When report cards arrived and the grades were good, we had in our hand evidence that we had excelled, had accomplished something that was valued.

Upon arrival in the workplace, however, we find that excellence is the expectation—the only expectation.

In nursing, or any other profession for that matter, one of the hardest things to accept is that often no one notices when we excel. This is very disappointing for us, since we have grown so accustomed to our families' praise. You may get to work every single day on time, but no one is going to commend you, give you a star, or brag about you.

Getting to work on time is the expectation.

It follows, then, that in the work world, you have to provide your own incentives. I know people who sit around and complain that no one appreciates them. "No one ever tells me I'm doing a good job," they moan. "No one ever notices if I take the extra time to do a better job or not."

So, as with the training wheels when we were learning to ride our bikes, we have some choices. We can make no effort to excel whatsoever, leaving the training wheels on the bike. Or we can try it without the train- ing wheels, fail, and immediately put the training wheels back on as we bemoan the fact that "I'm too afraid to try it again."

Or, we can try and succeed and when no one notices, we can just quit riding the bike altogether. That seems to be the worst pos- sible fate.

You have to weigh the option and make some decisions about how to get the positive feedback that you need—that we all need—to keep inspired and happy in our work.

I suppose you could take your mom to work with you. Every time you started an IV or took a blood pressure, she could run up and down the hall with you, patting you on the back and telling anyone who will listen how gifted and talented you are.

Or you can be your own cheerleader, a much better option. You can tell yourself what a great job you did. You can take yourself out to dinner for a really inspired job or reward yourself with a new garden hose. I never just buy household items because I need them. I always say to myself, "I deserve this new soup ladle. I've had a really busy week and I did a good job. I'm glad to have this new gadget and I deserve it."

Each day you live can be a burden to be endured or a gift to be enjoyed. Your ability to appreciate yourself and excel in what you do is just like everything else in life—it all depends on attitude.

So don't wait around for your boss or your coworkers to notice how wonderful you are. Tell yourself everyday how lucky they are to have you.

Shake your head in wonder as they fail to notice how truly special your talents are and just chalk it up to their inattentiveness. Make your own happiness. Be your own cheerleader.

The more you revel in your own successes, the more your patients and coworkers will benefit from being around someone who is happy in the job and takes pride in the work. The more you take pleasure in achieving, the more your family will benefit from a mom who likes herself or a dad who feels good about what he is doing in life.

In my opinion, there is nothing in life more important than being happy and sharing that happiness with others. I believe that is one of our greatest challenges.

So take off your training wheels and learn to enjoy how truly special you are. You'll not only feel better, but all along the way, you will be a better nurse.

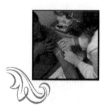

CHAPTER 12

HOLIDAY DUTY

A necessary but dreaded duty for most nurses is working on Christmas, Thanksgiving, and other holidays. These traditional family times make being away from home a double hardship, but most nurses attend to their holiday duty with a mix of joy and resignation.

First, we realize that if nurses hate to be away from their families on holidays, then patients must feel even worse. Being in the hospital during the time of traditional family gatherings make illness and recovery even more difficult. Many people push themselves to try to be home by Christmas. People who are admitted during the holiday season pin their hopes on being home before festivities begin.

Second, most of us just incorporate holiday duty into our family lives, especially in regard to our children. They are used to hearing that we have to work on weekends sometimes, so they know that mothers and fathers have other responsibilities. Saving lives and caring for sick people is a serious and important matter.

Even young children of nurses can understand that what their parents do is very important and sometimes entails some sacrifice, like having to wait until Mom gets home to open presents or having an evening Thanksgiving dinner so Dad can eat with the family.

Finally, we rely on our reminiscence of wonderful on-duty holiday stories. Many involve the sharing of the holiday meal. One nurse told me that when she and her cohorts saw the holiday schedule and learned that they were working, they decided they would try to spread a little cheer. They brought in a turkey dinner with all the trimmings for the families in the waiting room.

Another nurse told me about working in England during the holidays. Since the patients tend to stay longer in the hospital there, the families get to know the nurses well. During the holiday season, the families prepared feasts and brought the whole family, distant and near, to the hospital for a holiday meal. While it was hard to be away from their own families, the nurses loved the generosity and fellowship of families who were expressing gratitude to nurses for giving of themselves to benefit their loved ones.

Nurses have joyful stories, like the happy moments of babies born on Christmas Day to grateful parents who enjoy the greatest gift of all. Nurses also have sad holiday stories.

One nurse who worked with oncology patients many years ago related an experience she remembers vividly. She looked me in the eye and told me the exact date.

"I worked with leukemia patients," she said. "[Back] then, they almost all died. It was the days when hospitals were less user-friendly, and children were strictly banned from visiting. I [was caring for] a 32-year-old man who was dying of leukemia. I asked him what he wanted for Christmas that day and he told me that all he wanted was to see his children. I made a decision I have never regretted."

She went on to relate how she arranged with his wife to bring their three small children to the hospital the next evening. After her strict, rule-enforcing supervisor made rounds, she signaled to the stairwell for the wife to bring in the kids.

She went in his room a few minutes later and found all three children in bed with their dad who had the biggest smile she had ever seen. They showed him pictures, talked about Christmas presents to come, shared those precious moments that only happen between dads and their kids.

The patient died quietly the next morning with his wife at his side. Many years later, my friend is still profoundly moved by this experience. Nurses truly do touch lives.

I want to thank my colleagues who give so selflessly of their time and talent during the holidays. It takes a special person to be a nurse. Like our brothers and sisters in the military and the police officer and firefighter ranks who are on duty 365 days a year, we serve because we care. We care about people we don't even know. We care about people whose religion and skin color are different from our own. We care about people whose language we can't understand. Whether it is an important holiday or just a regular Tuesday, nurses are on duty everywhere doing what they do best: caring. Thanks for always being there.

CHAPTER 13

DOES YOUR FAMILY GET LEFTOVERS?

No, this chapter is not about dinner tonight. I just wanted to ask a pointed question about the significant relationships in your life.

A friend once related the story of an elderly gentleman she knew who was in the hospital. He was very ill and eventually died. His family was so pleased with the wonderful care he received while in the hospital; they went on and on about how caring and compassionate the nurses were. These nurses tended his needs with gentleness and seemed sincerely concerned about his comfort. They also took time to keep the family informed, to let them talk about this wonderful man's life, and to cry with the family when he died.

I had feared that this type of interaction might be a thing of the past in the current healthcare environment, but this family painted a picture of nursing as I pray it can always be.

My friend's story ended with this question: How can nurses expend so much emotional energy with their patients and then have anything left for their own families when they get home?

We all know how busy we are these days. No question, life is complicated. The "I'm busier than you are" contest is not our imagination; it's real. With increasing responsibilities, sicker patients, more demands for non-clinical activities, and the technology explosion, nurses are expending more physical and emotional energy than ever.

After a day of sharing the anguish of the ICU or emergency room, the intensity of the birthing room, or the challenge of the reha-bilitation unit, how do nurses go home and have anything left for their families?

A few responses are possible:

a. We have conditioned our families not to expect any emotional support from us. Sadly, emotional commitment may be one of the casualties of our current hyperactive lifestyles.

b. We just keep reaching down into some unknown emotional storehouse and just keep on giving. If so, will we run out or burn out some day?

c. As professionals, we have perfected the art of balance. We give of ourselves on the job and at home in equal abundance without compromising our physical or mental health.

I hope you have selected the last option. I think nurses are pretty smart. Most of us get into nursing because we are caring individuals who genuinely like people. One of the perks of the job is our ability to get involved with people on a personal level. A common workplace complaint of nurses is that the workload does not allow them to provide the kind of care they believe the patients deserve. That type of care almost always involves an opportunity to offer emotional as well as physical support.

Please take a moment and see which of the responses fits you. If you are overspending your emotional allotment and feel like you are burning out, I urge you to reassess your situation. If job, family, and other commitments are draining you of all of your physical and emotional energy, you will soon be useless to all of them as well as to yourself. Take some time for yourself. Allow yourself to heal and replenish your energy supply. Get some mild exercise and take some time for yourself. Don't wait until it is convenient; it never will be.

If you are short-changing your family because you are overextending your emotional capabilities on the job, stop for a minute and weigh your priorities. Childhood is a fleeting gift that goes by very quickly. Don't miss this in your children. Aging parents will not always be there, so appreciate them while they can still enjoy your attention. Significant relationships need care and nurturing, just like a plant, or they will wither and die. So save some strength to put some effort into your own personal needs.

Am I asking the impossible? I certainly hope not. No one can take advantage of you without your permission. If you are overextended at work, you are allowing it to happen. I do not want you to short-change your patients who need you so desperately, but I believe we have enough care and compassion for both patients and family. We just have to hit our stride, to find our balance. I encourage you to take control of your situation and be sure your family is not getting leftovers. They deserve the best.

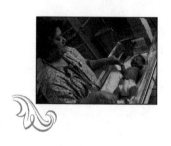

CHAPTER 14

PONDERING—
A VANISHING
ART

"Where do I want my career to be in five years?"

"There ought to be a better way to provide discharge instructions than when the patient is walking out the door."

"What is the true meaning of life?"

When is the last time you sat down and tried to address issues such as these or answer a truly puzzling problem? How long has it been since you just sat quietly and tried to solve a daily dilemma? Thinking about a question while you are driving in rush-hour traffic or running from patient to patient does not count. When was the last time you really sat and pondered? I bet you can't remember.

The art of pondering is being undermined by the hectic pace of living in modern society. With new technology and breakthrough scientific discoveries, however, it seems that pondering has become more critical than ever. We still need someone to ask serious questions. "Is all this technology causing more problems than it's solving?" "What's happened to our leisure time?" "How are we going to deal with the aftermath of health problems caused by increased productivity and less relaxation?" In the face of all of the new technology and increasingly complex machinery, nurses need to take a step back to assess themselves and their own work settings.

Can you remember a day when you did not have a fax machine? Of course you can. But can you imagine living without one now? No; the fax has greatly simplified so much of our daily workload. Nevertheless, we did manage to get things signed, sealed, and delivered before we had fax technology.

How about those other labor-saving devices which were supposed to simplify our lives—the cellular phone, pager, copier, computer? Is your life, in fact, simpler because of them?

These wonderful technological advancements have increased our productivity, but they definitely have not simplified our lives. In fact, they have allowed the workload to increase. They have made us more accessible after work hours. They have shrunk the world so that the once-distinct lines between work and rest are either smudged beyond recognition or completely obliterated.

What healthcare costs will we pay for this increased productivity? The costs will be high. We work harder, sleep less, study more, exercise less, and eat more poorly than any generation before us. We are caught up in a whirl of activities that threaten not only our work lives, but our very existence.

In an effort to improve our possibilities of survival, I propose that we spend more time pondering. Here are a few suggestions:

♦ Engage in the time-honored tradition of the bubble bath. Block out 30 minutes of time at least once a week. No cell phone, no pager, no papers, nothing. Just you and the bubble bath. Soak in the warm water and think about all the good things in your life. Ponder your good fortune, family, and health. Do not let negativity barge into your reverie. Just relax and enjoy. This simple act will add spring to your step and help you appreciate what a wonderful life you are living.

♦ Solve perplexing problems by pondering. If something is bothering you, some patient is just not reacting like you planned, or some part of your life is careening out of control, take a few minutes to open yourself up to your creative power. We humans have a wonderful ability to think and problem-solve. The catch is a lack of time and interest in actually searching out the options. Go someplace where you will not be disturbed. (Closets and bathrooms are often good options for personal timeouts.) Devote just a few minutes to focus on one specific problem and envision possible outcomes. Then make your best decision and implement it. This simple act can take only a few minutes, but it can be very worthwhile. The key is to give the situation your absolute attention, and then unleash your best creative genius to find the best solution.

♦ Ponder just for the fun of it. Sometimes, we need to ponder situations just to be glad they are not our responsibility. Imagine how your city would look if you had been the one to design the transportation system. Ponder the changes you would make if you were the CEO of your institution. Think about your life if your first child had turned out to be quintuplets. Pondering those types of problems will make you glad to be you.

We have such rich innovative minds in healthcare today. We are great problem solvers. My fear is that our increasing reliance on technology will cause us to overlook the greatest technology of all—our own creativity.

Dedicate some time to the disappearing art of pondering. Today's healthcare problems need the creative genius of all of us.

CHAPTER 15

BEING IN CHARGE

While many nurses are born leaders and love the challenge of being in management, today's nurse managers are caught between those making decisions and those doing the actual work. Frequently, the nurse manager has the unenviable task of implementing the views and plans of administration with little or no input. This process may mean leading the staff in a direction they prefer not to go—"working leaner and smarter," which, restated, means doing more with less.

When the staff on the unit sees the daily problems of trying to save money by cutting corners, they take their concerns to the nurse manager. The manager is then faced with the challenge of translating those concerns into a language that decision-makers will hear and understand. A further problem results when resources are economized, while the planners seek to maintain the same or higher levels of outcomes. When outcomes slip—such as patient satisfaction and timely discharge from the hospital in a state of improved health— the blame is usually aimed at the mid-manager rather than at those who set the cost-containment strategies in motion in the first place.

Another issue for the nurse manager is the responsibility for producing results with a team of someone else's choosing. Although numerous nurse managers are involved in selecting the actual persons hired for the unit, other entities set the staffing budget that dictates the level and pay of these employees. When hospitals try to economize by replacing professional nurses with unlicensed, undereducated assistive personnel, the challenges for the nurse manager multiply. Delegation of activities to unlicensed personnel is an important responsibility for nurses, and the nurse manager knows the problems that arise when the mix of licensed and unlicensed personnel is changed.

Given these hurdles, one might ask why anyone would want to be a nurse manager in today's chaotic healthcare environment. The answer stems from the quest of professional nursing itself. During their educational preparation, nurses are taught the scientific process: examine the situation, ask questions, gather data. In order to drive their decisions, nurse managers must make plans based on the data. When nurses do make decisions, they are and should be accountable for outcomes. Finally, nursing education is based on the ability to evaluate actions and determine what works and what needs to change. These activities, known as leadership and problem-solving, are the basis for managing a nursing unit, a hospital, a city, or a country. Nurse managers have the opportunity to practice nursing in its purest form, and that challenge along with the stature of leadership are the driving forces behind nurses choosing the management role.

Some nurse managers have become quite successful at giving feedback to administration to affect and change the healthcare climate. They are learning business rules and jargon, how to talk about outcomes in terms of cost and productivity. In fact, having seen patient complaints and injuries increase, many hospital administrators are listening to the advice of nurses in the management ranks and are rethinking the policy of replacing registered nurses with unlicensed personnel.

Nurse managers have also learned the business side of healthcare. Unfortunately, an initiative cannot always be implemented simply because it is the best thing for patients. Healthcare is a business. Nurse managers, however, have learned how to integrate being businesspeople as well as nurses, bringing a human and caring side to the cool, dispassionate business decisions that are made every day in hospitals. Benefits have been felt by the hospitals, the patients, and the nurses themselves. Nurse managers tackle the challenges of healthcare by relating to the grassroots level because they were once there, and they advise advocating at the administrative level where the decisions are made. Maintaining this balance is a tightrope that requires skill and dexterity, but in the long run, nurse managers are first and foremost nurses. Their passion for high-quality patient care makes everyone's job easier.

CHAPTER 16

DEALING WITH REALITY

I recently saw a nurse throw up her hands and declare in an angry, tear-choked voice, "Why in the world did I ever get into nursing?"

She had just learned she was getting two newly-admitted patients. She already had more to do than she could possibly handle in this lifetime, and she knew it. Call it a sign of the times—doing more with less, too much work and too little time, stress, burnout, anger, despair. Is there any hope?

Of course there is always hope, but how do we manage these frustrating situations? You've heard of *attitude adjustment*. Then you may be ready for an "expectation adjustment." We were all idealistic and zealous when we became nurses. What happened?

I am wondering if we can boil it down to an expectation/reality mismatch. It goes something like this: We expected to have time to listen and learn what was really bothering the surgical patient with two little children at home. We expected to make a real positive difference in people's health and happiness.

The reality, however, is that patient teaching occurs during the four minutes while you are administering your evening medications, when you really need to be paying attention to right patient, right dose, and the other "rights." The reality is that the only one who listens to the patient's worries about not being able to care for her two small children is the housekeeper. The reality is not what we expected.

So do we try to change our expectations or do we try to change the reality? One thing you learn about nurses very quickly is that we do not lower our expectations for our patients. The idealists in us are alive and well. We work to achieve the ideal, whether it is optimal health or a peaceful, dignified death. But I would like to offer a suggestion about our expectations of ourselves.

For some reason, nurses think they are invincible. We think we can and must do everything better and more quickly than anyone else. Faster is better, right? I also have watched the corporate world similarly speed up with some resulting angst and burnout. However, let's face it. In the corporate world, if the two columns on the audit sheet do not add up, no one dies.

Dealing with life and death situations is the factor that skews our vision. Just like police officers who deal with critical situations, we become consumed by the nature of our work. We lose focus of the fact that not every decision is life and death. If a patient quits breathing, we react immediately and decisively with the full force of our physical and emotional selves to save a life. Unfortunately, when the announcement comes that the parking lot is being repaved and we have to find alternate parking, we often react the same way. We expend a lot of energy over decisions which are not worthy of the adrenaline drain they trigger.

Perspective is the key. I stand by my sure-fire way of deciding how much energy to expend on any situation—the five-year test. Before you invest your precious time and energy in any situation, apply the five-year test: Am I going to remember this in five years? We each have only so much energy, so let's save it for the truly worthy occasions. Energy depletion is a major reason we feel the stress, burnout, anger, and despair mentioned earlier. We are just too tired to deal with it. So, anything that saves our energy is bound to make our lives a little bit easier and less hectic. Applying the five-year test is an easy way to save time and energy for the really big decisions.

Chances are good that if you give the wrong medication and have a disastrous outcome, you will remember it forever. So, medication administration is a situation worthy of your time and energy. The parking lot situation, however, is not. Yes, it is an inconvenience, a bother, just one more thing; but chances are good that it will **not** become a vivid part of your history. Accept what you cannot change and park somewhere else. Don't worry and fume over it.

One more thing—the pace of healthcare has accelerated. We cannot slow it down or stop it. We cannot control the demands others make of us. But we can control the demands we make of ourselves. If you are not going to remember it in five years, move on. Make a decision, don't second-guess yourself, and leave it in your rearview mirror. Take care of yourself. Nurses are a precious commodity.

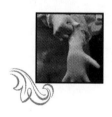

CHAPTER 17

NEW BEGINNINGS

Beginning something new? What a wonderful feeling! The promise of success or happiness is right there, just out of reach and yours for the taking.

Do you ever notice the thrill of anticipation when you begin a new book? You open the cover and move anxiously to the first page. Anticipating the unknown is such a delicious feeling! Once you have read the book, even a few chapters, the course is set and the end may even be predictable, but ah, the act of beginning the journey holds so much promise.

I believe each new day and each new year holds the same promise. The dawn of a new day, a new year, or a new century gives us an opportunity to look back at our successes and to look forward to our opportunities.

Anyone not expecting that each new day will be far better than the last may find they have unknowingly predicted the future. If you don't expect to find happiness, then everyone who is working to make your life better is in for an uphill battle. Ultimately, most of them will finally give up, your expectations will be met, and you will be miserable.

So, the primary rule for having a happy life is, "Expect it to be happy." This expectation then raises the question, "What do nurses want or need in order to be happy?"

When we look at the progress professional nursing has made over the past 200 years, we realize we have truly come a long way. Where we used to stand up when a physician entered the room and did as we were told, we now take an active partnership role in managing the care of our patients in hospitals and our clients in the community.

What will the future hold for nursing? I hope we resolve to be more inquisitive, more intuitive, and more intelligent.

◆ *Inquisitive*—Seeking new challenges and exploring innovative ways to do our jobs better are lofty goals for nursing. The time is right! Nurses are finally beginning to see a life beyond the hospital walls. We are inquiring about better ways to serve the public in nurse-managed clinics that promote wellness and delay infirmity. We are getting bold and innovative in our efforts to seek funding for those ideas that are not based on the traditional medical model but on ideas that prevent illness and promote a better quality of life. We are inquisitive, we ask questions, we seek new ways of doing things. Just because it has not been done before does not deter us from trying it.

* *Intuition*—That gut feeling an idea will work, that this patient is just not responding well, or that something is missing in the treatment plan is a hallmark of nursing. Although nurses have been served well by intuition, we have traditionally treated it like a secret handshake, only acknowledging our successes to each other. In the new openness of modern healthcare, however, it has become proper to discuss things we cannot explain scientifically in healthcare. Chaos theory, holistic health, complementary therapy—all of these concepts have opened the door to the possibility that there are things that

nurses do that simply defy explanation. I am eager to see nurses gain confidence in our intuitive sense and our nurturing prowess. Intuition is a gift that we use in our practice every day. Now we may be able to talk about it and help others develop their own suppressed intuitive powers.

* *Intelligence*—Nurses excel in the ability to think critically and make sound decisions based on knowledge. We can achieve high quality in nursing only if we have the knowledge, and knowledge is changing at a rapid pace, just like everything else in this world. Nurses must value continuing education, read more, keep up on the latest technology, and take individual responsibility for improving the knowledge level in nursing. We need to demonstrate our thoughtful impact on healthcare, so the best and the brightest of the next generation will see nursing as a viable and desirable career option.

I urge you to savor the tingling excitement and anticipation of each new day and new year. I hope you are blessed to savor all of the wonders and joy each new day brings as we make every life we touch just a little bit better.

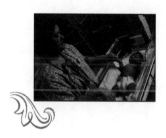

CHAPTER 18

REACHING BACK INTO YOUR PAST

I always tell nursing students to be nice to all the nurses they encounter because they will be bumping into them for the rest of their careers.

The family of nursing is quite small and intimate if you stop and think about it. We all revolve around the same core of operations—healthcare. The chances of running into old friends and acquaintances are pretty good if you continue in the nursing profession and get around a little.

Take a minute to think back to those nurses who have truly touched your career. We all have those people who shared some of our most glorious, and some not so glorious, moments of our careers. A few stand out, such as my nursing school colleagues who helped me sort through dirty laundry after I dropped my new engagement ring down the laundry chute in the pocket of my critical care isolation gown; my first head nurse who patiently listened to my novice ideas for "fixing" her nursing unit offered during my second week on the job; and the nursing supervisor who sat with me in a conference room and restored my shattered confidence after my first medication error.

Now, answer this question: When is the last time you talked to one of those people so instrumental in the formation of your career?

We drift into our own worlds, get busy with family and career, form new friendships and ties, move to different parts of the state or country, and somehow never get around to reconnecting with those voices from our past.

"Well, why should we?" you might ask. "That was then, and now is now. Why bother to look back?" I know many people who do not like reunions because they are reminders of the past and seem to have little relevance to the present. I would offer the idea that our present is a direct reflection of our past, whether we like it or not. Even if your past is something you would like to forget, I still believe it guides your daily actions. At the very least, our mistakes give us a direction to avoid.

In addition, reaching back into your past can have the following benefits:

* You will make someone feel good (happy, important, relevant, connected). Just the fact that you would take the time, energy, and expense to call sets a positive tone for this action. Everyone feels good when other people take the time to notice them.

* *You* will feel good. Face it, you do feel good when you do something nice for someone else.

* You will contribute to the historical bond of professional nursing. We nurses are a family, whether we like it or not. That is the beauty of a family; you get along with some better than others. You may fuss with some, but through it all, your family is a support that is always there. We need to work on this historical bond in nursing, both in nurturing it as well as in recording it for nurses who come after us.

* You might just rekindle a friendship that will bear fruit. You never know when you might need a reference, a new job, or a collaborator on a project.

So, how do I find the contact information for these old friends? That may take a bit of detective work if it has been a long time. However, with the Internet, it is easier than you think. There are many free search engines which will seek names, addresses, phone numbers, and e-mail addresses with just a little bit of information. If you have a name and a city, you will probably succeed. Seek information from colleagues. If your friend from the past was an OR nurse, ask someone in the local Association of Operating Room Nurses chapter if they know him or her. Call your old school or hospital and see if they can help.

Try reaching into your past and touching someone who had a positive effect on your nursing career. Who knows, maybe someone will reach out and touch you.

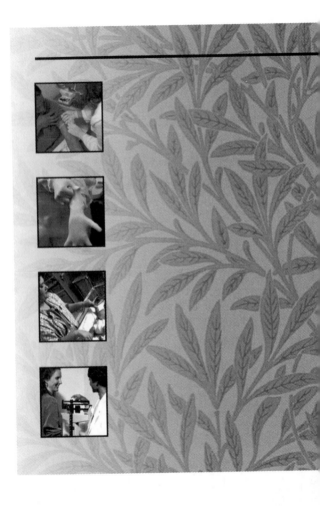

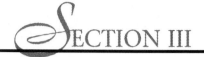

SECTION III

ALL THE
NEWS THAT'S
FIT TO PRINT

Serving the public is a major focus of nursing. Nursing remains one of the public's most trusted professions. This section focuses on the relationship of nurses and patients, that special bond that forms when a caring person is entrusted with the most intimate aspects of another human being. Nurses deal with life and death, pain and suffering, hopelessness and fear on a daily basis.

CHAPTER 19

I NEED A HUG!

"Hours and hours of tests!" my friend moaned after a day at the hospital. "I was exhausted and nearly in tears, afraid something was really wrong with me, and I missed an entire day of work. I was at the end of my rope." She went on, "Then a most extraordinary thing happened. The nurse who had been with me all day just gave me a big hug. Not only that, but she hugged my equally frustrated husband as well."

My friend reported that this magical moment made all the difference in the world to both of them. The fear, the physical demands of all of the tests, and their frustration were gone in an instant. Another human being had touched them, and their entire attitude was changed.

I pondered this simple act in relation to the fact that my friend was reporting on a day of tests in a healthcare environment. I would have expected a full report about her medical condition or questions about the tests and other informational things that people usually seek from us, their nurse friends and neighbors, but no. The first and only thing she chose to share was this spontaneous act of a caring nurse who recognized a desperate need for human contact . . . and provided a hug.

In light of the evolving political and social environment in this country, I have remained attuned to the fact that nurses are still allowed to touch. As it happens, we are one of the last remaining bastions of legitimate touch.

In the school, the workplace, the White House, and even the church, unsolicited and spontaneous touching has become an occupational hazard—a punishable offense.

For nurses, touch has always been a traditional intervention, a communication mechanism, even a therapy. We have made therapeutic touch into a credible healing modality.

So, what are the implications of this touch factor that so impressed my friend?

I submit that being allowed to touch is both a privilege and a necessity that brings with it great responsibility. Nurses have always assumed and welcomed the nurturer role. We provide for our patients with the assistance they would provide for themselves if they were physically or mentally able. If the patient cannot take medicine, we administer it; if the patient cannot breathe, we maintain mechanical ventilation; if the patient can no longer sustain life, we offer support to a peaceful death.

Working from a broad knowledge base, we assess the patient and intervene only as much as necessary to assist toward restoration of health. This might mean standing by while an elderly patient slowly and painstakingly feeds herself so she can be more independent instead of simply taking the easy way and putting the food in her mouth for her. It also means assessing when the patient needs human contact in order to feel connected to the world, to feel that someone cares, to avoid the chill of loneliness.

The reason nurses are still allowed to legitimately touch is that we use touch to benefit the recipient instead of ourselves. We use touch just as we use many therapies, an ice pack, fetal heart monitor, or thermometer. We have assessed the patient and found what, in our judgment, is needed.

I applaud that astute and caring nurse who recognized that my friend was nearing the breaking point and provided just what she needed: a hug!

I salute every nurse who takes a few minutes from a busy day (and they are all busy these days) to give the distraught patient a back rub at bedtime to ease away the tension of the day. This simple act not only provides comfort but also a human touch that promises that tomorrow will be a better day.

As we are inundated with more expensive high technology, more computers to make our lives easier, more unlicensed personnel who act as nurse-extenders to make our time go further, I implore nurses not to lose physical contact with our patients.

We are almost the only ones, outside the family, who can still legitimately hug our patients. We must protect and defend this

truly human and nurturing privilege that we
use so effectively.

CHAPTER 20

THE NAKED TRUTH

I want to talk about the bare naked truth about being bare and naked. I've given this topic a lot of thought.

Have you ever thought about why we wear clothing?

If you watch television, you might think that clothing is becoming optional. . . or at least minimal. In our society, however, clothing continues to have a lot of importance. Clothing protects us from the elements, adds to our beauty, and demonstrates our social position to the world. Wearing a designer trademark may catch another's eye and dressing sloppily may earn some critical looks. Clothing is very important to most of us.

So what about being naked?

A friend once told me about a hospital experience she had. She was in for same-day surgery. After she was taken to a rather large room for preparation, she was asked to remove her hospital gown so they could shave her. Since everyone knows that you have no dignity or choices in a hospital, she did as she was told.

"They stood me in the middle of this large room, stark naked, and proceeded to shave me. People were coming in and out, but I stood, naked as a jaybird," she wailed. "I felt like a side of beef!"

Now I am betting you could stand Miss America naked in the middle of that room and those same people would enter and exit without any more interest than just getting the abdomen shaved and germs eliminated. My friend didn't care about that, however. She was embarrassed, upset, and unforgiving. Her surgery went very well, but I had to ask about that. All she really volunteered was her humiliation and horror at being naked.

One of the things people find mysterious about nurses is our acceptance of the human body and our willingness to touch people. Our total comfort with bodily functions and ability to cleanse other people's bodies are a source of bewilderment to many. Most of us never give it a thought. We know that the bath is the best assessment opportunity of the day. We feel compassion for the older adult who can no longer control bodily functions or do normal hygiene. We take seeing people naked and touching people's bodies pretty much for granted.

Patients, however, do not come with this mindset. I don't care what you see on television, modesty is still a prized commodity for most of our society. People want their privacy respected and their bodies covered. However, a hospital is often an unlikely place for modesty to be a priority.

I think most nurses try to be very aware of patients' desires for modesty and their discomfort with having strangers look at, or touch, their bodies. I see nurses stop and pull the covers back over confused patients whose thrashing or turning has dislodged the sheets. I've seen nurses get someone to stand behind a patient so his gown won't flap open as he transfers from the wheelchair to the bed. We earnestly try to protect our patients' physical and mental health, as well as their personal pride, while they are in our care.

I would just ask that nurses continue to be aware of our patients' need for modesty. As we strive to do more with less, as we have to work quicker and smarter, I hope those shaping today's healthcare environment don't overlook the patients' need for respect and consideration.

Our patients know that their very lives are in our hands. Let's be sure they know we value that life by showing them the same courtesy we would want shown to us. We need to keep them covered as much as possible. Let's take the extra minute to shut a door or ask a visitor to leave or get a sheet to cover a patient's helpless nakedness.

The human body is a beautiful thing, and so is the human spirit. Let's be sure we nurture both in the patients we serve.

CHAPTER 21

IS "CARE" JUST A FOUR-LETTER WORD?

"Nurses care about patients.' What does that really mean?" my nurse colleague asked me during a discussion.

We were pondering what a caring encounter really was. Nurses care; that is why we are so vital to the healthcare team. It does not mean that others do not care, but we think we care in a special way. Our entire practice is built around the concept of caring.

Then, one of my colleagues asked the question that stopped the discussion in its tracks: "Can a nurse give good nursing care if he or she does not really care about the patient?"

Immediately, the chorus chimed in with a resounding "No!" He then asked, "Have you ever had a patient that you did not like?"

Well, the truth is, all of us have had patients that we do not particularly like. We promise to render safe and competent care to our patients, not to become their best friend. In fact, one of the wonderful things about nurses is that we are so good at what we do that most patients we don't like certainly never know it. After all, we care for bank robbers, child abusers, pushy mothers-in-law, and egocentric, overbearing corporate executives. Health problems are not reserved for the kind at heart. So, even though I gave the people I did not like good care, did I really care about them?

My astute colleague pointed out that there was a difference between really caring about someone and simply "tending" them. You can meet their physical needs, you help them on the road to recovery, you anticipate their needs, but do you really have to form an emotional bond with your patient to be a good nurse?

To be honest, I don't know. I want to say that I form an emotional bond with all of my patients, that I care about their lives and families, that I would do anything to help them on the road to recovery, but that would not be the truth. I probably would not donate my heart or my brain to any of them if they just spontaneously asked one day. My patient who asked for my phone number so she could call me if her alcoholic son beat his pregnant wife again made me wish I had never asked about how her family was doing, but I gave her the phone number anyway.

A lot of research is being done on what it means to care in nursing. As we strive to identify those things that make up a caring encounter and make us the caring profession, I think we must look equally honestly at those times when we don't care *about* the patient, even as we provide excellent nursing care.

You know, it takes a lot of energy to care. If you have ever had a baby, you know that those little bundles of joy are in need of constant care. We know that if they are denied a loving, caring person with whom to bond during those first precious years of life, they may have problems in later life.

So if patients enter into a caring transaction with us, what is our obligation? What do they expect from us? If we give good service, if we meet their needs, if we "tend" them well and to the best of our ability, have we lived up to their expectations or our own?

What do you think about a caring encounter? Do you have to care about every one of your patients in order to care for them adequately? As human beings, nurses have feelings about the people we meet. As nurses, we must rise above those feelings to offer excellent care in a nonjudgmental way to each and every patient. We are nurses; it's what we do.

Maybe I am the only one who has ever taken care of someone I did not really like, but I find that hard to believe. I think that nurses are caring people who look past the superficial things we don't like to see the person who has needs. We meet those needs.

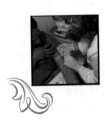

CHAPTER 22

PATIENT FEARS

I walked through the ICU one day. One patient appeared to have a dozen IV bags hanging and the usual body systems monitor with the cardiac rhythm in plain view. He was on a respirator and had a couple of other machines that I must admit I did not even recognize. I watched the nurse working in that environment, so relaxed, capable, competent, in control, so aware, so ready. It was magical—a scene of total confidence as this very sick man let this nurse hold his life in her hands. I was awed.

Then I looked again and tried to imagine how this scene appeared to someone who was not a nurse: his wife, his children, his friends. It was probably frightening, the first time they saw someone they loved relying on so many machines, so many bags of medicine. And, I am willing to wager that it probably scared them every time they visited him.

For one thing, all that equipment is a reminder of how sick a critical patient is. It is a reminder of just how fragile life can be. But another aspect of their fear is that this scene is foreign, strange, very complex, and monstrously intimidating. It must be somewhat akin to how I feel when my car will not start. I look under the hood and feel total intimidation and bewilderment. Nothing looks familiar except the radiator where the water goes. Almost everything is unknown to me and causes fear that my ability to get to where I am going depends on something I cannot fix. Family members of patients in the ICU must feel that way about the cardiac rhythm strip—it looks familiar from seeing it on television, but they don't know what it means.

Fear must be constant when people are in the ICU. Fear of the unknown, fear of unwanted outcomes, fear of being unable to fix everything. ICU nurses have grown particularly adept at addressing the fears of visitors and patients over the years, but it remains a challenge.

How about the simpler things in hospitals as they relate to patient fears? As we get busier, I worry that we are forgetting the natural fear that patients and families have of the everyday things we do. We used to go into the patient's room *without* the nasogastric tube to explain what gastric suction meant and how it was done. We would explain in simple terms and let the patient ask questions. *Then* we brought in the equipment and in a soothing, soft voice explained every step of the procedure. We stayed with the patient for a few minutes until calmness had returned.

In these hectic days of doing more with less, I wonder whether we still have the time to leave the tube behind, to recognize and allay patients' fears.

How about a simple blood transfusion? Today, people are terrified of having someone else's blood pumped into their veins. They are afraid of the idea, the procedure, and the potential outcomes. I wonder if we recognize that fear and try to reassure the patient; or if we feel lucky to even find the 10 minutes it takes just to get the paperwork done in order to get the blood delivered and the transfusion started?

Of course, it's easy for me to sit at this keyboard and preach about the need to spend quality time with our patients, to take time to reduce their fears and promote their comfort. I haven't just worked 11 hours, my feet don't hurt, and I am not worried that I might get a call in the morning to work for someone who is out with the flu.

The realities of nursing today are sometimes grim. But I have to hand it to nurses. I still see nurses laughing, caring, explaining, and talking gently and soothingly to frightened patients. You just cannot get a good nurse down. Even when nurses are tired and frustrated, we still take the time to recognize and allay patients' fears of the unknown.

I think that nurses know that things always get better. We have problems, crises, even disasters—but things always get better. Sharing that ray of hope and confidence is what makes a frightened patient feel the security and confidence that everything will turn out well. I guess when you spend your life taking care of people who are helpless and often hopeless, you insulate yourself against sadness and despair so you can continue to function. The current healthcare crisis is sad and discouraging, but nurses continue to function. In fact, when things get tough is when we often rise to our finest hour.

I know that nurses will continue to make a difference in people's lives. I hope you will remember that our everyday environment can be a hostile and frightening place for patients. I implore you to find the time to answer questions about procedures and spend a few moments just being present to your patients who trust you enough to place their lives in your hands. Healthcare can be a fearful place to patients; nurses make it safe.

CHAPTER 23

CULTURAL DIFFERENCES AND NURSING CARE

Society appears to be tiring of discussions focused on culture or multiculturalism. And yet, the facts are simple: We are different. We come from different places. We've read from different books and had different experiences. We've heard different lectures and had different role models.

Some people place value labels on these differences. Deciding on these values, or "judging," creates an atmosphere in which we do not seem to get along very well at all.

Those of us who have spent the greater part of our nursing careers working with various ethnic groups are equally aware of the differences. But we continue to see the value of peace and harmony, and we have gone on with our work in spite of a society that is color, class, and gender conscious.

I would like to respectfully and humbly share with you a few hints that have helped me enjoy my nursing career, working with many people who are different from me.

♦ I have always gone into each setting, no matter how different from my own culture, expecting to be welcomed and accepted. I firmly believe that whatever you expect is what you will find. I expect them to like me, and I expect to like them and to enjoy my nursing experience with them; and I usually do.

♦ Focus on the ways we are alike, not on the ways we are different. I value the confidence Hispanic elders have in their *curanderas* (faith healers). I admire those elderly black women who spend many hours on Sunday morning and into the afternoon celebrating their love of God at church. I may not do those things, but they do. However, the majority of the things they do are exactly the same things that I do. They worry about their kids. They wonder what to fix for lunch. They try to lose weight. They enjoy fresh flowers. They try to make their money last to the end of the month. So do I. We are all much more alike than we are different. Most of our problems between races, genders, and age groups start when we focus on how we are different.

♦ Understand that racism, sexism, and ageism are not exclusive to any one race, any one gender, or any one age group. It was a shock to me to learn that elderly people are sometimes biased against teens or younger people. I have found that racism runs across all races as well. Some people do not realize that multiculturalism includes the culture they are biased against as well as others. When I saw racism and ageism across many groups, I learned an important lesson. Bigotry is not part of anyone's culture. It is a learned personal flaw.

♦ Learn about other cultures **and** share yours. People love to talk about areas in which they have some expertise, and nothing makes an expert like living an experience. So, go on. Ask people about their culture. I've noted that nursing students are fairly comfortable with this aspect. When I ask them, however, if they share their own culture in return, they look at me as if I have suddenly grown two heads. Don't assume that others know your culture. Share your experiences, too.

♦ For example, ask this question about your patient's culture: "What did you eat for Sunday dinner when you were growing up?" Black beans and rice as a response from a patient may sound strange to me, but my patient may be equally surprised to learn that my family had fried chicken every Sunday of my youth. It was just a hard and fast rule at our house. Now, most people cannot even remember the last time they actually fried a piece of chicken. Sharing how my values and customs have changed over the years, however, shows yet another area where we share more than we differ.

♦ In general, always, always do what you do best—be a caring nurse. The language of caring is universal. When you bring love of people and a sincere interest in their well-being into any setting, culture does not matter. You will succeed.

CHAPTER 24

DEFINING WHAT IS ACCEPTABLE

The public is understanding and accepting when they think of nurses handing a healthy newborn to an eager mother. They look kindly on the caring nurse who soothes the pain of an elderly woman with a broken hip. However, some have a harder time when they think of nurses dealing with those patients who have communicable diseases, who are unpredictable, or who are unpalatable, such as criminals. Nurses don't get to pick and choose the cases we take; we are called to care equally for everyone, even those who may be considered less than desirable.

How do nurses deal with universal acceptance? To answer this, it is important to realize that nurses have to accept many things in
our profession that non-nurses would find it
difficult to accept, to say the least. What
nurse has not heard someone ask, "How can
you stand the blood?" or say, "I can't bear to
see anyone suffer." We take these things as
normal parts of our jobs.

We also care for people who some in society
label and judge simply because they are different. In today's enlightened healthcare environment, we might think that such prejudice and
narrow-mindedness are a thing of the past. But
I remind you that there are nurses today who
are uncomfortable taking care of people
they label "different." It is difficult to be nonjudgmental in our care. We have standards,
principles, and feelings just like everyone else.
While we may have negative personal feelings,
as professional nurses, we still are called to provide quality care to everyone.

How do you feel about taking care of
someone who is gay, who has had an abor-
tion, who is a prostitute, who is a drug addict
or an alcoholic? I know nurses who do not
want to care for patients who have attempted

suicide because it clashes with their belief systems. I know nurses who prefer not to work with AIDS patients because they are uncomfortable and maybe a bit afraid. I know nurses who dread the idea of caring for a patient addicted to alcohol or drugs or someone with a sexually transmitted disease because it offends their moral standards.

HIV-positive and AIDS patients tell us they can sense when a nurse or healthcare provider is afraid of them or resents caring for them. What a tragedy to be dying of an incurable disease and then be rejected as a person, too.

I am reminded of a defining moment in history that I was privileged to watch. It was the handshake that shook the world when Princess Diana visited a London AIDS hospital and actually touched a person with AIDS. Those of us who had worked with AIDS patients realized the enormity of that small act that reverberated around the world.

On a daily basis, nurses do things that might be difficult for other people to do. We see and touch, we hear and feel the unthinkable. It is unacceptable that children die, but we see it. It is unacceptable that vibrant young men lose the use of their limbs, but we share their anguish. It is unfair that family members die and leave grieving loved ones, but we stay and absorb some of the shock and despair. We face the unacceptable every single day, and we rise above it. That is what nurses do.

I hope that nurses never allow their willingness to care to be based on society's definition of who deserves care and who does not. The one and only thing that is acceptable to us is to render professional nursing care when and where it is needed.

Regardless of who the patient is or what the health problem, nurses are there. Whether the patient lives in a palace or under a freeway, nurses accept the fact that help is needed and give it willingly. I salute all of you who bring the true meaning of acceptance to life every day.

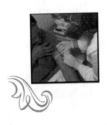

CHAPTER 25

EMPOWERING OUR PATIENTS—A NEW MANDATE?

The public is thinking about health in new ways. Current political and public sentiment, stemming from the tobacco settlement and the AIDS epidemic, has focused on personal accountability. And, in this new day of limited resources and personal accountability, nurses must help patients think and do more for themselves.

For nurses, however, this concept is not new. Popular media outlets are defining the idea of personal accountability as becoming knowledgeable about promoting healthy behaviors and preventing illness. In fact, nurses have *always* seen their role as working with the patient and family in health promotion and disease prevention. Our comfort level with this "new" responsibility is much greater than those who have always simply told people what to do and expected them to do it.

Yes, I admit that patients used to stay in the hospital for two weeks after back surgery and now stay only approximately 48 hours. In the old days, nurses did more for patients because patients stayed in the hospital longer. I respectfully submit, however, that nurses did not then nor do we currently control when patients actually enter and leave the hospital; physicians and insurers do. We did our job then as effectively as we do now, and it was the same job—empowering the patient and family to be optimally healthy.

Nurses have traditionally said, "You start preparing the patient to go home on the day he or she arrives at the hospital." We've always believed that it was therapeutic to foster independence in patients since they go home without the nurse in constant attendance.

We urged and even coerced patients out of bed only a few hours after surgery, often against their wills and better judgment, because we knew the alternative of lying still was much more dangerous for their health. We used our pain control techniques to minimize their discomfort. As we did so, we were teaching them what we were doing so they could manage their own care effectively at home. I propose that we were empowering them to care for themselves in our absence, just as stipulated in the mandate of today.

A fertile opportunity for empowerment today is in our vulnerable populations. In elderly and indigent populations, the predominant theme has been more paternalistic. We give money (e.g., Social Security, Medicare, and welfare) and in return, they buy what we tell them to and go to the hospitals we select. Could it be that constantly being told what to do regarding health has carried over into a reluctance or inability to take positive steps to change unhealthy behaviors in these populations?

For example, we know that low-income persons view their health more pessimistically and are more likely to report an external locus of control, i.e., doing something for their health because someone told them to instead of doing it spontaneously.

Many health-delivery models are now admitting, however, that vulnerable populations can and do make sound health decisions when given the information and options to take positive measures. Nursing has many examples of community-based clinics in low-income populations where positive outcomes are happening every day. Elderly men and women are forming walking clubs, taking nutrition classes, lowering their cholesterol levels, and insisting that their health needs be addressed. Many opportunities exist for nurses to take the initiative to empower vulnerable populations to make sound decisions. The healthcare market has changed to offer them options not previously available.

I urge all nurses to take an active role in sharing the joys of health empowerment with all of our patients, particularly our vulnerable populations. They will feel better, and so will you.

CHAPTER 26

INDEPEND-
ENCE DAY

Independence. What does it really mean?
Some people see it as being able to do what
we want when we want . . . most of the time.
Others may see it differently.

In any case, it might surprise some people
to know that fostering independence is an
important function of professional nurses.

For example, nurses who work with the
elderly understand just how important the
gift of independence can be. In fact, I would
go so far as to say that gerontology nurses are
every bit as interested in function as they are
in health. Function, what the patient can and
cannot do, is the vital link to independence.

Those of us who work with the elderly
know that they usually pray for good health,
but what they tell us they value most is being

able to stay in their own homes. It does not matter if that home is a palace or a shack, it is one of the most valued parts of an older person's identity.

One of my fondest nursing memories is of an elderly patient with diabetes who had only one leg. She was fighting eviction from her run-down, two-room home of over 40 years. In a wheelchair, she could no longer maintain the dilapidated shell of a house and, having a very low income, she could barely afford her insulin. However, she refused to leave her home.

"It may be a shack," she said through tears, "but it's my shack and I'm staying here!" In spite of her trials, she had received the gift of independence, which she treasured and was unwilling to give up.

Are we surprised? Wars have been fought over this concept, even in our own country. Isn't it strange then that when a country is "struggling" for independence, the world stands in admiration and often supports the cause? When a little old lady begs for independence, however, we label her "stubborn" and find legal ways to "save her from her own foolishness."

I often wonder where our zeal to take elders out of their own homes and put them in group facilities "for their own good" comes from. Certainly it is easier for families if they do not have to worry. It is easier to care for these elders if they are all in neat little rows of rooms. It is easier for the government to watch over its money if they only have to deal with a few overseers rather than a large number of people. But every one of these rationales make life "easier" for someone other than the elderly person.

A further consideration is the fact that the majority of the elderly in this country are women.* I often wonder if we would be as eager to usurp the independence of the elderly if three fourths of them were men instead of women.

Nurses face special challenges as they work with elders, both men and women, whose healthcare needs increase with age.

---

*United States Census Bureau, Special Populations Branch, Population Division: Population by Age, Sex, Race and Hispanic Origin, March 2000. Available at: http://www.census.gov/population/socdemo/gender/ppl-121/tab01.txt. Accessed April 6, 2002.

Nurses have a special role in safeguarding the independence of the elderly. We must guard against taking the easy and convenient way out just because it makes it easier for us. Particularly important is the tendency to step on the elder's right to independence in the name of health and safety. When we say a person cannot stay at home alone anymore because it is unsafe or unhealthy, we must be sure we have exhausted every plan, no matter how inconvenient the plan might be, to allow that elder to keep the gift of independence.

Sure, it is easy to recommend a nursing home, moving in with a daughter or son, moving into assisted living far from the old neighborhood. It often seems like the best solution. The elder is safe, secure, cared for. After all, what is giving up a little independence to have a longer and safer life? The answer is that it is no problem at all, unless it is *my* independence you are sacrificing. Then it gets personal.

I invite all nurses who are involved in these types of decisions to let it be personal every time. Think about how you would feel if your own independence was threatened.

Explore all of the alternatives. Take the time to discuss the situation and personal preferences with the patient. Foster the gift of independence if at all possible. To all of our patients, particularly the elderly, it is one of the greatest gifts we can give.

CHAPTER 27

POWER STRUGGLE

Power—it seems like a crazy idea to discuss something such as power in this text, when nurses feel like they have so little of it. However, aren't nurses faced with power struggles every day? Who wins in these cases? And more importantly, are we prepared for these struggles?

Power implies that someone has control over someone else. Let's identify who nurses control and who controls us. Then we can decide whether the struggle is worth the effort.

Patients are perhaps the least powerful persons in the hospital, the clinic, or even in their own homes when faced with a healthcare worker. Of course, institutions tell us that the patient is the most important person in the hospital, the reason for our being there, our customer. None of us will argue with that logic, but I still believe that even in the most enlightened, customer-friendly institutions, the patient has almost no power.

We tell our patients when to get up, when to eat, even what they can eat, when to get out of bed, and when they can go home. We "restrain" patients whose safety is in jeopardy. We tell 30-year smokers that they cannot smoke in our hospitals and they cannot leave—all for their own good. Then we give them drugs to make our control of their smoking behaviors easier to manage.

A vital part of our control over patients is in pain management. Patients do not get pain medication without some input from a nurse. By our charting and our collaboration with physicians, important decisions about pain management and other therapies are made every day.

We are experts at controlling families and friends. We tell them where they can park before they even get in the hospital. We tell them when they can visit and how many can come in a room at one time. We also have the ultimate source of control over families and friends: information flow. We can tell them or not tell them whatever we choose.

Nurses, however, are also controlled by other people. Ancillary departments, for example, exert great control over nurses' schedules. If a patient is going to have laboratory work done from 9:00 AM until noon and will be in physical therapy all afternoon, the assessment, bath, dressing change, and other nursing needs must consequently be done before breakfast.

Physicians exert control over nurses by virtue of the nature of the relationship between nurses and physicians. Most actions in hospitals, clinics, and home health locations are dependent or interdependent. That means that nurses do not perform the actions without a physician's order. Examples include medication orders or the application of heat or cold.

Hospital administration also controls nursing actions by instituting the staffing patterns that directly affect the nurses' ability to do a thorough, professional job of assessment or teaching. Administration controls costs, supplies, personnel, and policies.

So, on the one hand, nurses exert great control over powerless patients, and on the other hand, we are highly controlled by various other persons in the healthcare setting. How do we balance this chaotic approach to our daily schedules?

I believe we all understand the importance of using our ability to control in a helping way, never simply for the pleasure of being in control. When we make decisions that put us in the position of controlling the behavior of others, we must always be sure the decision will benefit them. We must never let our own frustration with those who control us interfere with our judgment regarding the decisions we make for our patients. No matter how tired or frustrated or angry we feel, we have to always remember that patients put themselves trustingly in our care. We are bound by duty, morals, ethics, and law to treat them with dignity and professionalism.

Power is an awesome responsibility. Nurses respect the power we have. We need to use that power to make patients safer and healthier in all clinical settings.

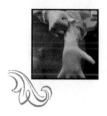

CHAPTER 28

ATTITUDE IS EVERY-THING!

In my speaking opportunities, one of my favorite topics is attitude. I love to share the Family Circus cartoon in which Billy and Dolly are both contemplating a rose. With a scowl, Billy grumbles at the fact that roses have thorns. Dolly, however, gleefully sings her happiness that thorns have roses!

At the bottom of this cartoon, I have written the words, "Attitude is everything!" I keep it prominently displayed on my bulletin board for my students to ponder.

It seems strange to me to have to tell someone that attitude is important. It seems so self-evident, it may be ridiculous to even mention.

But if that is true, why do we encounter so many people with bad attitudes?

I no longer give the benefit of the doubt in this matter. I used to say, "Oh, she is just having a bad day," or, "I must have caught her at an inopportune moment," or some other excuse. Not anymore. I do not excuse and cannot tolerate bad attitudes. Life is too short and the world is too needy to have to tolerate someone who is diligently working to make things worse. I simply have no patience for these bad-attitude people anymore.

In healthcare, a positive attitude is vital. You cannot realistically expect sick people to always have a happy outlook or a positive attitude. Therefore, the attitude of the nurse is even more vital to a healthy outcome. Be careful, though! An over-the-top bright and cheery approach is not the answer either. Sometimes, too much cheer is as bad as too little. The answer here, then, is in a basic expectation that things will go well.

Nurses must convey a positive attitude when working with our patients. We must expect that the patient will do well. We must share that expectation with the person and family. We must appear glad to be at the patient's bedside (whether we are or not), and that patient should feel like the most important person in the world because of our attention and caring. If we are complaining about being short-staffed, about being short-changed in the cafeteria line, or about how much we pay in taxes, the patient will be hard pressed to believe we really care about the situation at hand. An important part of the art of nursing is making the patient the center of our universe when we are rendering care.

A positive attitude is vital when working with other people besides patients as well. Coworkers have problems of their own, problems that you probably would just as soon not have to share. Your positive attitude, however, might just help them get through at least one shift with a little less stress and a bit more positive energy.

Another important aspect of having a positive attitude is its effect on your personal achievement. To get ahead in life, we all need a little help. Think about it. Recruitment and retention strategies occupy a large amount of the hospital administration's time. When they make retention or promotion decisions, it is just smart business to select the person with a positive attitude since that person will contribute to the type of work setting that makes people want to come to work and stay there. A positive attitude can be a career booster, and a negative attitude can be a career buster.

So, is attitude important? No—it is vital! A healthy attitude tells the world that not only do you like them, but you like yourself as well. There is no greater gift you can give than to make someone's day a little brighter. And the funny thing is, the more you give away happiness and kindness, the more it comes right back to you.

I challenge you to consciously go out today and make this world a little brighter. You will be surprised how good you, and others, feel.

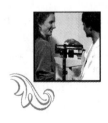

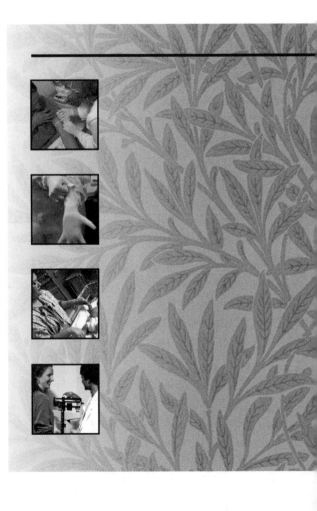

NEWSFLASH!

*W*here is the nursing profession going in the twenty-first century? This section allows us to take a look at where we have been and where we are going. The newsflash is the realization that nurses are in charge of their own destiny. What nursing will look like in the coming decades and who will be delivering nursing care is of paramount importance to the future of healthcare.

CHAPTER 29

THE GOOD OLD DAYS

What do experienced nurses talk about when they get together? They talk about the "good old days"! In truth, however, they may or may not be considered the good old days, depending on the selective memory of the speaker. But since the good old days are often used as a benchmark against which we measure our nursing world today, it is important that we view the past realistically.

I was eating a chicken hot dog with a slice of tomato on it and one of the new fat-free potato chips one day when it dawned on me that all of the foods on my plate tasted exactly the same. I suddenly realized, I was not savoring the taste of a hot dog. I was savoring the memory of the taste of a hot dog. Let's face it. Hot dogs have not tasted like hot dogs since

161

we discovered cholesterol and took all of the fat and sodium out of them.

Okay, so everything is starting to taste the same. So what we taste is what we remember tasting when we grew the tomatoes in our backyard or picked the beans out of our gardens.

I began to think of nursing in those same terms. Yesterday and tomorrow are always better (or worse) than today. When we look back at how things were in hospitals in the 1970s, we remember more help, lower acuity, nicer supervisors, and while the work was hard, it was never impossible.

Today we are understaffed, patients are sicker, supervisors manage by a computer formula that has little relation to the human situation, and the work has gotten more difficult to manage. Many nurses are burning out, and some are leaving the profession altogether. What has changed from the good old days? Or are we just viewing the past more favorably than it really was, making today's challenges appear more overwhelming than they really are?

Actually, nothing has changed. Back then we were tired at the end of a shift. We doubled back and worked double shifts to cover. We worked short-staffed. Our patients were not as sick, but our technology was not as sophisticated. We did not have all of the ancillary help we do today, such as respiratory therapists and physical therapists, but the patients did not have all of the therapies ordered back then either.

We still had to give a lot of medications, but the Physician's Desk Reference was thinner. Emergency rooms had no physician on duty most of the time, but it took so long to get people to the hospital that most of the really critical ones died before they got there anyway.

We had new drugs in the 1970s; chemotherapy was just beginning and there was great fear of these killer drugs. We had devastating illnesses; the word "cancer" meant a death sentence. We had social problems too—our young men were coming home in body bags from Vietnam. Yes, we had our problems then, and those problems seemed overwhelming—just like they do now.

I submit that things weren't really all that different "back then." In hindsight, things always look better or worse than they really were. Did hot dogs really taste that good when they were packed with all sorts of unhealthy ingredients? Or does it just seem that way?

Instead of lamenting about how much worse things are now under managed care, we nurses need to spend our precious time and energy making today better. Some things are worse, but many things are better. If we focused as much of our time on solving problems as we do on grumbling about them, there would be no problems left to solve.

It is so easy to complain and whine. It takes almost no effort to point out what everyone else is doing wrong. But to offer solutions to problems takes effort. You actually have to think about the problem. Then you must create some alternative solutions in your mind and think through each one, weighing the pros and cons. After all that effort, when you finally arrive at a possible solution, you have to not only *share* it, but you have to *sell* it to others. Selling or convincing others takes time and energy. Then there is always the risk that they will buy the idea, and it might fail.

Most nurses will just take the easy way out and complain. We would rather be part of the problem than part of the solution. Is there one nurse out there who would trade places with Florence Nightingale caring for desperately wounded soldiers on a dirt floor? Of course not! We take the advances in modern nursing for granted and tend to focus on what still needs to be done.

That focus is great if we see these needs as challenges and rise to meet them. But if we use the shortfalls as excuses not to try, then the next generation of nurses will pay for our complacency and inaction. What a terrible legacy we would leave if our unrealistic memories of the past prevented us from striving to make tomorrow better than today.

The "good old days" can only be good if they make today and tomorrow even better.

CHAPTER 30

FAME AND FORTUNE

Why did you become a nurse?

Think back to those months, years, or perhaps decades ago when you made that decision. What was going through your mind?

I'm betting most of us will say something like, "I wanted to help people," or, "I wanted to do something that made a difference," or, "I like people and I wanted to ease suffering." I also bet that none of you said, "So I could get extremely rich and retire at age 40," or the equally unlikely, "So I could be famous and have everyone ask me for my autograph." No, most of us did not come into nursing with high expectations regarding the potential for fame and fortune. Most of us came into nursing for noble and people-centered reasons that benefit our patients every day.

I would like to ask one question, though. Where is it written that helping people must be accompanied by poverty or obscurity? For some reason, most of us in nursing think that if we mention money or celebrity, we have committed some sort of dishonorable sin against the purity and goodness of the nursing profession. For some reason, we have a low perception of our value.

And yet, nurses frequently go well beyond the call of duty to help a patient, knowing that the benefit will be a payment made by an insurance company to the hospital with no recognition of the nurse. Furthermore, the physician is the person of record in regard to the patient's care. Nurses are the ones who are there night and day to assess patients' needs, ponder the alternatives, make the decisions, and carry out the plans to help the patients get better. The nurse also evaluates the care given and determines changes that need to be made to improve in the future. This activity calls for high-quality technical skills and above-average thinking skills.

Nurses contribute that vital link to health-care effectiveness. If the world did not have nurses, it would have to invent us! Therefore,

I think we need to get out of the victim mentality that has become so comfortable for nurses. We seem to feel the need to find someone who will speak for us instead of telling the world ourselves how valuable we are. We need to be innovative and creative in our approach to patient care and to expect that these activities will be rewarded.

As healthcare changes over the next decade, new avenues of care will emerge. Entrepreneurial opportunities will make it possible for nurses to compete for healthcare dollars in ways that improve health access and care for many patients. Nurses will be compensated and rewarded for using their critical thinking skills to manage the many healthcare challenges posed by the large baby boomer population. I hope nurses will value these contributions and will insist that others value them as well by seeking adequate compensation and control over practice. Patients will benefit when the creative genius of nurses is unleashed to improve healthcare delivery to wide varieties of patient populations.

Did you get into nursing to find fame and fortune? Probably not! But when it comes within your reach, grab it and make no apologies. Nurses are very special people. It is time we started acting like we believe it.

CHAPTER 31

STUDENT NURSES— INVESTING IN THE FUTURE

Now, an important topic about our future—nursing students. There has been a huge shift in the minds and hearts of nurses regarding student nurses over the past few years, from a positive approach to a more negative one. I think this shift has been unconscious and perhaps even unwanted. Nevertheless, this change in thinking is out there in plain view, and it needs to be addressed.

First, we all agree that being a nursing student is an enormous challenge. For years, nurses have welcomed their role in developing and mentoring students. It was a source of pride and self-indulgence to contribute in a meaningful way to a student's education. We looked at them as our future colleagues and perhaps our replacements as we moved on to bigger and better things. We also saw in them our own caregivers as we aged, so we selfishly wanted high-quality nurses who were almost as good as we were. Something, however, has changed.

Nurses who once were eager to have a student assigned to them now hide at the end of the hall, hoping not to be noticed when the instructor approaches. Even the most patient mentors are requesting limited time with students.

From all indications, nurses would rather just give medications themselves than watch a student prepare the drugs. Why? What has happened? Are today's students suddenly much less talented? Have the faculty stopped teaching?

Truthfully, it appears that students and the faculty have remained relatively the same. What has changed is the practice environment. Nurses are being asked to do more with less. We have all seen and heard discussions about this situation, but what does it really mean when it comes to student mentoring?

Doing more with less means caring for sicker and sicker patients on the general medical-surgical units, for example. Today's typical medical-surgical patient would have been a typical ICU patient just a few short years ago; but ICU is expensive, and the goal has become to get the patient out as quickly as possible without incurring high costs.

Doing more with less means attracting a decreasing number of unlicensed assistive personnel to the field who have less qualifications and abilities. And the reason? The computer industry is begging for employees who can read, write, and think—and it pays attractive salaries. We pay unlicensed assistive personnel low wages, ask them to do menial tasks, and often show them little appreciation. Many have moved on to greener pastures in other industries, leaving us short-handed in hospitals. This change in staffing mix means that nurses must often do low-skill tasks along with all of the other expected responsibilities.

Doing more with less means fewer nurses on each unit for consultation, collaboration, and support. Many hospitals have stripped nursing units to the bone in order to decrease costs. The result—a preponderance of poor outcomes, such as falls and pressure sores, linked to low ratios of registered nurses. Administrators are now hearing from more patients, families, and physicians who are becoming upset and frustrated with the situation. Therefore, hospitals are attempting to rectify this short-sighted action, but the return of nurses to the hospital is slow, and students are paying the price.

In summary, why don't nurses want to work with students? They are too tired, too overworked, and too busy. They have more than they can handle with their own patients and expected responsibilities. If time allowed, however, I believe most nurses still want to work with students.

Don't get me wrong. Faculty members have the obligation to prepare students to provide care. Students cannot learn solely on the job; they must know a great deal from laboratory practice before they ever set foot on the nursing unit. Together, however, faculty and professional nurses can provide a meaningful experience for the student and a safe experience for the patient; faculty must be attentive to student needs while nurses are attentive to patient needs.

We cannot give up on educating future nurses. We need them now more than ever; but this education is a cooperative process. Everyone—the nurse, the faculty, and especially the student—must take responsibility for making the experience effective. Tomorrow's healthcare system depends on it.

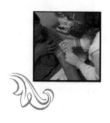

CHAPTER 32

GRADUATION —NURSING BEGINNINGS

Graduation from nursing school is a wonderful experience. Grateful relief that the rigors of the formal education process are complete and eager enthusiasm to begin a new career are just some of the emotions that new nurses experience.

A whole new crop of nurses emerges from the hallowed halls of nursing schools. They are a welcome sight. These enthusiastic new nurses join a tired nurse population. Nurses in hospitals, where most of the new graduates get their first jobs, are feeling the pinch of the nursing shortage, so each new class of graduates are welcomed with open arms by the current nursing workforce.

What will these new nurses find? Will they find a mentor who is happy to show them the ropes, to share insights, to offer support when the first problem arises? Or will they find seasoned nurses who are too tired to help, stretched too thin to offer the moral support they need, or who have the attitude, "I learned the hard way, now you learn the hard way."

I believe that emerging nurses are a fragile commodity. I think they must be handled with care. I can hear my experienced colleagues sighing under their breaths and muttering something about, "What makes them so special? No one gave me special treatment."

Many nurses have long memories. We remember every slight, every snub, every rude word that was ever uttered by a thoughtless supervisor or an abrasive colleague. We take it personally, and we vow to get even. Then, unfortunately, we often strike out at the person we view as dependent or less powerful than we are. That person is often the new kid on the block, the new graduate. At a time when they need nurturing and support, we often use

them as a way to get even for all of the grief
we have suffered over the years. It feels so
good to finally "get even." But I want to
point out the risk with this type of abusive
behavior.

Previously, if the new graduate could
not take it, they would leave. That way,
only the fittest and the strongest survived
in the busy hospital environment. It was
really not a problem; we would just get
another new student who was probably
stronger anyway. The problem is that
today, the applicant pool is diminishing.
There aren't long lines of other students
waiting for that job. If we run off the new
graduates who are somewhat insecure or
who fail to be assertive from the first day
on the job, we run the risk of having no
one to share the complex duties of the
work environment.

The environment that the new graduate
of today is entering is vastly different than
the one we encountered during our first
month as a new nurse. The patients are
sicker, the machines are more complex, the
pace is faster, and the supportive nurturing
colleague is harder to find. It can be over-

whelming. Professional nursing cannot afford to invest two to three years in the education of a nurse only to find that after a frustrating first year, this nurse decides to get into another field. When nurses leave, not one patient benefits. Other nurses suffer because they must now pick up the slack.

How can nurses present a compassionate and welcoming environment for new nurses? How can we assure that they will thrive and prosper in their new career?

Smile at them. Tell them you remember what it was like. Share some anecdote about how you did similar things when you were a new nurse. You are a hero to them, an icon, a person of such high esteem that they can never hope to be as experienced and competent. Let them into your real self. Invest a little time with them. I remember being scared to death, and I remember how much a reassuring smile meant to me.

We have to transform the nursing environment into a safe, secure, and welcoming place for new nurses, or they will go elsewhere to find one. When you invest in a new

nurse, you improve the future for both of
you.

CHAPTER 33

THE EMERGING WORK-FORCE

Worry seems to be mounting about the next generation entering the workforce. In particular, older workers are spending a lot of time worrying about how to manage these twenty-somethings because they are "different." They have different expectations and needs. Since some of these members of the emerging workforce have become our next generation of nurses, perhaps we should take a closer look at them.

It is important to point out some of the positive attributes of this young, emerging workforce. They are very goal-driven and out-come-oriented. They are critical thinkers who are optimistic and innovative. After all, they grew up watching Sesame Street! The "one of these things is not like the other" rhyme was their initial introduction to critical thinking.

They have great self-reliance skills, yet a fragile self-confidence. Because in some cases Mom and Dad were at work all day during their formative years, they tended to offer their children lots of positive feedback when they did get home. Members of the emerging workforce, therefore, can be accustomed to being told how wonderful they are and how everything they do is extraordinary. They like and want praise and motivation.

Now, they are entering a workforce where certain expectations exist. In this working world, interaction with supervisors tends to occur more often when things go wrong, not when things go right. Think about this one—when was the last time your supervisor complimented and praised you for dispensing your medications on time? You probably can't remember because this is the *expectation.* When we go above and beyond the expectation, we often get positive feedback, but not for simply meeting expectations.

Bradford and Raines, in their 1992 book *Twentysomething: Managing and Motivating Today's New Work Force,** pointed out successful ways to work with and manage the emerging workforce. Let me share a few of their examples.

◆ The emerging workforce "comes to us with poor skills, especially in math, writing, and communication basics." If the calculator breaks, they will have problems figuring their medication doses. Either encourage your organization to provide remedial help with math skills or be prepared to assist with medication calculations. Do so in an accepting way without showing scorn or indignation.

◆ "They are not team players and have little company loyalty. They want to know the 'why' of things they are asked to do." The

---

*Bradford LJ and Raines CM: *Twentysomething: Managing and Motivating Today's New Work Force.* Denver, 1992, Merrill-Alexander Publishing.

emerging workforce brings many positive attributes to offset these problems. They are extremely creative and outcome-oriented. If you explain what the goal is, why it is desirable, and challenge them to meet the goal, they will work tirelessly to meet it. They do not want to have someone standing over them telling them how to do it. Just explain the goal and get out of their way. They are great problem solvers.

◆ "The emerging workforce wants respect, recognition, praise, and time from their managers." The praise and recognition factors are the easiest and hardest things to provide. They cost nothing and are easy to give. However, in this fast-paced work environment, they are the first things to go because of fatigue and lack of time. It might be worth your time to invest a bit of effort into recognizing and praising your new colleagues. They will reward you by rising to your greatest expectations and perhaps discovering a better way to do things along the way.

Today's emerging workforce will be our caregivers tomorrow. They will be our replacements and our future. To ensure their effectiveness and longevity, we need to invest a bit of time and energy to understand them and to make them feel welcome in the healthcare environment. They will meet our expectations, good or bad. Expect them to be extraordinary; they will not let you down.

CHAPTER 34

YOUNG NURSES BLOOM WHERE THEY ARE PLANTED

Spring is a time for lush gardens of lovely flowers. A bountiful garden requires a certain amount of time and commitment, but it is a welcome sight for all to behold. Few of us approach the creation of a beautiful garden plot by driving to the nursery, purchasing seedlings at random, and then flinging them into the front yard to fall where they may. After several weeks of no nurturing or attention, would we be surprised that we also had no flowers?

However, this let-them-fend-for-themselves attitude often prevails when young professionals embark on their careers and enter that most sacred of places, the "real world." Just as seedlings soon die without proper planting, adequate water and nutrients, and some tender loving care, many new nurses are also left to "wither on the vine" for lack of adequate nurturing and positive role models. This withering may take the form of disillusionment and frustration, early burnout, or chronic underachievement. And as these bright, potential stars are lost, the nursing profession suffers from their absence.

Why should professional nurses who long ago "paid their dues" take the time to invest their precious energy and expertise in the development of new, inexperienced nurses?

From a purely practical standpoint, we have already invested in their education, and we may need their assistance in the future.

Almost every nursing program receives some type of federal and state funding. Student tuition and fees cover only a fraction of the actual college costs to educate any future professional. Nurses pay taxes. Therefore, we are subsidizing every nursing student who attends school. When we fail to nurture them early in their careers, we are throwing away the money we have invested.

What about planning for the future? The graying of the nursing workforce is a reality as the average age of nurses increases with each passing year. Many who enter nursing schools today are older, second-career students. Obviously, we do not have enough young nurses to replace those who will retire in the next 25 years, just in time for the profound effects baby boomers will have on the healthcare system in the United States. It is in our own best interests—and that of this society—to nurture and mold our neophyte nurses into the most competent and confident care professionals possible.

And what about professional duty? It is the hallmark of a profession that it maintains a mechanism for self-perpetuation. To sustain our current number of nurses, educational institutions continue to produce new graduates, who are prepared with entry-level skills. It is, and always has been, anticipated that much of their education will occur on the job as they mature into true professionals. If we wish to be recognized and paid as professionals, we are obligated to act professionally. An important aspect of that role is to nurture our new nurses.

A final reason for contributing to the success of new nurses is that it is simply the right thing to do. If we expect new graduates to come into our nursing units and contribute in a positive way, we must offer them insights into why we do things and how we learned what we know. We must share and show them how to excel at their chosen work. If we do this, they will follow our example.

In summary, if we expect novice caregivers to be ignorant and unmotivated, if we choose to see only the things they don't know and their shortcomings, and if we believe they were put on this earth to make our lives totally miserable—that is exactly what will happen.

So I challenge every member of the nursing profession to make a contribution to the future health of the global masses. I ask you to take new graduates under your wing and treat them as you wanted to be treated when you were new. If we initiate a culture of benevolent sharing and caring, it will be handed down from one nursing generation to the next. And when we are elderly and in need of caretakers, we will benefit from the time and energy we expend today. Just as a beautiful bouquet is the reward for tending a flower garden, a confident nursing workforce will be our reward for investing time in our new nurses.

CHAPTER 35

LIFELONG LEARNING—A NURSING COMMITMENT

Lifelong learning is one of the hallmarks of the nursing profession. While it is a challenge, it is also a commitment that never ends. Nursing's goal is to promote a growing grasp of knowledge and to offer the public the benefit of the very latest innovations. A vital piece of effective health promotion in the public arena is a knowledgeable and competent nurse.

Continuing education for nurses is usually defined as programs beyond the basic preparation which are designed to promote and enrich knowledge, improve skills, and develop attitudes for the enhancement of nursing practice. It's important to note that not all education takes place in a school setting. Nurses can learn from professional journals that report the latest findings. Many courses are offered in the community by private providers aimed at keeping nurses' knowledge on the cutting edge. Some professional organizations host continuing education classes in conjunction with their meetings. There are also home-study and on-line courses which enhance continuing nursing education. Finally, most healthcare facilities offer regular inservice courses that assist nurses in obtaining the latest information about healthcare delivery. Simply put, educational opportunities are everywhere.

How do you decide which continuing education programs to attend?

A fundamental strategy includes examining your career goals. Where do you want to be in five or ten years? If you like your current job and feel fairly secure, your continuing education courses should be aimed at making you more competent in the things you are doing now. Do not rule out other areas of nursing, though. Technology-based education that teaches you how to surf the Internet, how to e-mail and manage electronic databases, and how to use audiovisual programs will enhance your marketability in the workplace.

An additional strategy for enhancing your flexibility and making you more marketable to future employers includes learning about the areas in which healthcare is moving. So, even if you do not work in managed care or in politics, for example, continuing your education in nontraditional areas can help you in the future. Another example, completing a course in medical Spanish, might make you a more attractive candidate in a multicultural healthcare environment. Likewise, special expertise in bioterrorism might broaden your opportunities to contribute to nursing in other settings.

A popular trend in continuing education for nurses is retraining for different roles. A wide variety of new opportunities are opening up for nurses in community-based roles in home health, managed care, and health promotion, for example. For nurses who have been hospital-based for their entire careers, moving into the community can be overwhelming. Attending an appropriate continuing education course can be a positive way to prepare for this new challenge.

The alternative to lifelong learning is stagnation, and no nurse should settle for the status quo. Our patients expect the best; that is what they deserve. And that is what they get from professional nurses who make continuing education an integral part of their nursing careers.

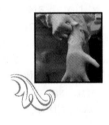

CHAPTER 36

CREATING CHANGE

Change is everywhere, and it is inevitable. Many people are averse to it; however, the idea of creating change is especially attractive in the nursing profession because it may be an answer to much of the unrest in our profession these days.

Nurses have always been quick to adapt to change, even though we usually have very little control over when it comes or how it affects our day-to-day patient care. Not too long ago, we came to work and found that all of the really sick patients had been rounded up and moved to a new central location, the ICU. Critical care specialists evolved, and patients' outcomes changed.

Next, we came to work and learned we would be drawing laboratory samples and performing EKGs ourselves. Administrators called it "total patient care." Nurses took on these additional responsibilities. We changed, even though the benefits to the patient were less clear.

In fact, we consistently find ourselves reacting to changes which are often ill-conceived and money-driven. If we could just orchestrate these types of changes ourselves to improve patient care, I am confident that the work environment would improve and patients would benefit.

Here are a few ways we can effect positive change:

◆ First, if you have an idea for a better way to do things, speak up. Briefly put your idea in writing and show how it will benefit patients and/or the hospital. Remember, satisfied patients are a desirable commodity, especially to hospitals. If you can contribute to patient satisfaction, your idea may have the "zing" to gain universal appeal.

◆ Second, volunteer to serve on committees that influence change, such as product evaluation and risk management committees. Of course, you may not have time to be on a committee; but if you don't serve, who will? The decision makers will be people who may not truly understand the needs and realities as you do. Be a part of creating change so it benefits both patients and nurses, as well as the hospital or agency.

◆ Third, know your rights. Employees have many legal rights under state and federal law. Your state nurses association is only one of the many resources available to help you understand your rights and ability to create change.

◆ Lastly, work with your hospital as a member of the team that creates change. Bringing the collective strength of the hospital and nurses together to make positive change is a powerful force. Use numbers and research articles to show your hospital how your ideas can be beneficial to everyone.

Remember, nurses are critical thinkers. We embrace change when it improves patient care. We are the patient care experts. I urge you to remember the one reason why patients come to hospitals or home health agencies in the first place: nursing care. They can get everything else they need at different locations. Patient care is the sole reason they come and the reason we are there. Let's use

202

our knowledge and our concern for our patients to create change that benefits everyone.

CHAPTER 37

THE HUMAN SIDE OF TECHNOL-OGY

How can anyone be against technology? After all, more people are alive and thriving because of modern technology. We save tiny babies, aged adults, and severely injured persons because of the new technological advances in medical science. How can anyone not value saving lives? However, I must ask this follow-up question: Have *all* of the outcomes from technology been good for nursing and healthcare?

I don't think so. With all of the advances that are supposed to make our lives easier (i.e., faxes, copiers, cellular phones, e-mail, videoconferencing), why aren't our lives any easier? In fact, I would go so far as to say that our lives have become quite a bit more difficult and complex with all of the countless modern conveniences of today. What happened?

Today's modern technology has allowed us to have everything at our fingertips in a matter of seconds. We are saving lives that just a few short years ago would have been lost. And yet, it appears to me that the mood in hospitals has grown more intense and grave than ever before. Why aren't we happier about our new modern conveniences?

In my opinion, with the advent of managed care and the rapid advances of modern technology, we find everyone trying to do more with less. Of particular concern, we find fewer nurses caring for sicker patients. Let me explain.

First, rapid advances in technology make keeping up with new equipment a daily challenge. In past years, we could go to a couple of inservices and one good conference each year and know everything that was important about our specialty area. Today, new equipment and modalities emerge almost *daily*. A huge percentage of our time is spent in keeping up-to-date on new equipment. This is a must; a responsible nurse knows how to use the equipment that is available to benefit all patients.

Second, a fast-growing healthcare phenomenon today is the long-term acute care hospital (LTAC). These hospitals contain patients who were traditionally on the medical-surgical floors of hospitals just a short decade ago. They have been moved here because the medical-surgical floors are now filled with the ICU patients of the 1980s. These patients have been moved from the ICU because the ICU beds are filled with patients who would have been dead 10 years ago without the advances in technology today. Our patients are sicker than they've even been before.

Finally, much like our counterparts in the corporate world, we are doing more with less. Nurses are the largest personnel pool in any healthcare institution, so when economic indicators demand cuts, the first place the ax usually falls is in the nursing pool.

In summary, I propose that the new era of technology has certainly benefited nurses and the way we do our jobs. However, we must continue to adamantly advocate safe patient care within this new era, as we attempt to do more with less. We must use technology and all of its advances to help us do our jobs more effectively.

CHAPTER 38

A STROLL
DOWN
MEMORY
LANE

And so we are nearing the end of this book. I hope it has helped you to smile as you reminisced. I hope you have been able to recapture some of the passion and wonder you brought to nursing when you were just starting. I hope it has given you a glimpse of the wonders you will share over your career. Looking back and looking forward are all part of keeping balance in our nursing lives.

Look back to times when there was no nursing shortage. Life was simpler back then, at least I like to think it was. Look back to times when there were nursing shortages. Nurses kept right on serving the public, just as they are doing now.

I have talked a lot in this book about the unique aspects of nursing that fascinate non-nurses: seeing people die, touching and bathing people, dealing with blood, acceptance of naked bodies and naked souls, dealing with difficult people, crying with families. I hope you laughed as we talked about humor in the hospital, and maybe you cried as we talked about how nurses deal with their own grief.

Which of the chapters was your favorite? I think I liked best the chapter dealing with the concept of human touch; I mentioned that nursing is one of the few remaining professions that can legitimately touch other people. The awesome responsibility of that gift given to us by society continues to inspire me to be judicious and caring any time I touch a patient.

I also loved writing the chapter about using humor in nursing. I don't think we use humor enough. It is a terrific stabilizer and coping mechanism. When times get rough, humor is often the first victim when it should be the last. The best thing that happened when that column originally appeared was the feedback that I received from nurses about how they used humor in their own hospitals and work settings. One hospital radiology department sent me a photo of their Halloween costumes they wore to work, all depicting various radiology tests. They were clever, tasteful, and hilarious. I am consoled to know that humor still lives in hospital settings.

Perhaps my favorite topic has been how nurses treat other nurses, especially students and new nurses. Nothing makes me any angrier than to hear the phrase, "Nurses eat their young!" I absolutely refuse to believe or accept that. If it is true anywhere, then shame on that nurse. I think that all of us need to be reminded about how it feels to be new, to be unsure, to be scared. Nurses, who excel at easing the pain and fears of a first-time surgery patient, should do no less for a first-time nurse. And so I have discussed the importance of nurturing other nurses, especially those new in the profession. If one new nurse has stayed because of something you said or did, then congratulations to you.

I have tried to point out that everything in life is about attitude. If we expect to be good nurses, to have a happy and fulfilling career, to serve others in a way that makes them healthier, to lead toward better healthcare for all—if we expect to do that, we will. Attitude is a choice. You can choose to have a positive or a negative attitude, and your life and career will be whatever you expect it to be.

I wish for each of you a positive future as a nurse. Take care of yourself; don't wait for someone else to do it for you. Know that you are appreciated by me and every other nurse who realizes the sacrifices you make on a daily basis. I wish health and happiness for every one of you in your personal and professional lives. I am happy to share these *Stories for Nurses: Acts of Caring*—there is much to share.

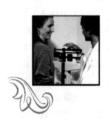

CHAPTER 39

A VISION FOR NURSING

How has professional nursing evolved to its present state? Do you wonder if there was a great master plan? Are we exactly where great thinkers thought we would be 30 years ago? Or, have we just happened?

If we want to make nursing better in the future, we must take control; we must have a vision of nursing in the year 2020 and create a viable plan for reaching that vision.

I believe our vision must be one that focuses on nurses at the forefront of health—health delivery, health promotion, health maintenance, and health restoration. I see nurses as the leaders of healthcare, the access and departure point for every health need for every patient. Much like physicians were in the 1980s before managed care fragmented access and care, I think nurses should be the gatekeepers of healthcare.

We must have a vision where ancillary groups, such as physicians, healthcare institutions, private insurers, and special interest groups, support the work that nursing does to keep people physically and mentally healthy. Nurses have to focus on our public health, mental health, and health promotion prowess to become the nation's primary healthcare provider of choice.

No one should enter or leave the gated community of health delivery without a nurse who is responsible for their primary healthcare before, during, and after their encounter. This responsibility should be in collaboration with the patient. Nurses should approach each member of the public in a partnership role for optimal utilization of health services. We can certainly call on our ancillary services if our patients need brain surgery, gait training, or in-hospital care for a few days. However, the promotion, management, and restoration of their health should be a nursing responsibility, guided and controlled by one nurse.

We must have a vision in which nurses partner with insurers and government entities to provide health services in a more cost-effective way. The savings related to reducing and managing pain, decreasing rehospitalization, reducing recurring chronic problems, improving the quality and quantity of life, and restoring dignity to the dying process are all nursing-based savings opportunities.

Nurses being seen as the nation's primary healthcare provider of choice, the gatekeepers of healthcare—now that is a vision.

Nurses partnering with government and private insurers to provide health promotion, maintenance, and restoration—that is a plan.

Once we have established this shared vision for nursing, ideas and strategies will begin to take shape. Pediatric nurse practitioners will find solutions to the problem of uninsured children. Geriatric nurse practitioners will take charge of the nursing home industry and fix it. Women's health will focus on the natural aspects of menstruation, childbirth, and menopause instead of making them medical problems. Complementary therapies will decrease the over-dependence on pharmaceutical agents currently experienced by so many elders. *Health* care will replace *illness* care.

Once the benefits of being educationally prepared for a clear role as the gatekeepers of healthcare have been clearly articulated, under-educated nurses will reenter the nursing education system and prepare for their future roles. This infusion of new students will increase nursing educator needs, resulting in higher salaries and inducing younger nurses to choose education as a career option. And, if the current educational systems do not meet the needs of the emerging workforce, they will be replaced with newer on-line, user-friendly educational approaches for preparing nurses for the vision of our future.

The future of nursing is ours. If we grasp it, we will thrive. If we timidly decline to get involved, we will be left behind. Someone else will rise to claim healthcare and move it in their direction. If we miss this opportunity to be the shapers of the future of healthcare, the quality of patient care and the nursing profession itself will suffer.

What is your vision for nursing? I challenge you to move forward and make professional nursing better than it is now. The future of nursing is too important to be left to chance.

INDEX